Table Of Contents

Dash Diet Snacks and Appetizers Recipes 29

Dash Diet Fish and Seafood Recipes 39

FREE GIFT!

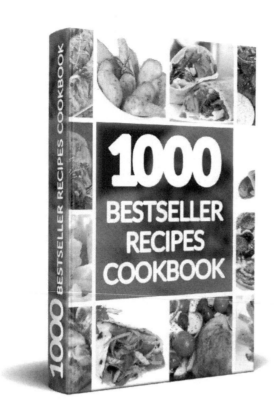

In order to thank you for buying my book I am glad to present you
- 1000 Bestseller Recipes Cookbook -

Please follow this link to get instant access to your Free Cookbook:
http://www.bookbuying.top/

Introduction

Your new life starts today! You will become a healthier person and a much happier one!
Are you curious to find out how you can achieve that? Well, it's actually really simple!
All you need to do is to start following a dash diet.

We know that the word "diet" frightens you but things are different this time.
This dash diet is nothing like the others you've followed before! This particular diet doesn't forbid you from eating your favorite foods!
Do you want to find out more about this special and easy diet? Then, let's discover together what this diet really means.

The dash diet is actually called The Dietary approaches To Stop Hypertension.
It might sound a bit pretentious but it basically means that you must start consuming more healthy foods and fewer fats and sodium.
During a dash diet, you get to eat nutritious foods that allow you to prevent the appearance of hypertension and other similar conditions.
Everyone can benefit from a dash diet and it's up to you to make it your lifestyle starting now!

Here are some main guidelines to help you understand what dash diet is:
1. You should reduce the consumption of salt to a maximum of 2300 mg/day.
2. You should consume more veggies, fruits and low-fat dairy products.
3. You should reduce the consumption of bad fats and other products that contain a lot of cholesterol.
4. You should pay attention to how much sugar you consume and you should replace regular one with brown, palm or coconut one.
5. Consume whole wheat products.
6. Consume less alcohol.
7. Exercise at least 30 minutes per day.

As you can see, the dash diet is very easy to follow!
So, why don't you opt for it today?

Once the dash diet is part of your life, the only step you need to take next is to purchase this incredible cookbook.
It will help you get started with your new diet and it will allow you to make the best dash diet recipes in the world!
So, what do you think?
Are you ready to start this amazing journey?
Have fun!

Incredible Pumpkin Pancakes

These pancakes will make your day a lot better!

Preparation time: 10 minutes
Cooking time: 10 minutes
Servings: 4

Ingredients:

- 2 tablespoons baking powder
- 3 teaspoons cinnamon, ground
- 2 and ½ cups whole wheat flour
- 2 teaspoons ginger, ground
- ¼ teaspoon cloves, ground
- ¼ teaspoon nutmeg
- 2 cups low fat buttermilk
- 2 eggs, whisked
- ¼ cup olive oil
- 1 cup pumpkin puree
- Cooking spray

Directions:

In a bowl, mix nutmeg, flour, baking powder, ginger, cloves and cinnamon and stir. In a second bowl, mix oil with buttermilk, eggs and pumpkin puree and whisk well. Combine the 2 mixtures and stir well. Heat up a pan over medium heat, spray some cooking spray, pour ¼ cup of the batter, spread and cook until it's done. Flip, cook until your pancake is golden and transfer to a plate. Repeat with the rest of the batter and serve your pancakes right away. Enjoy!

Nutrition: calories 254, fat 3, fiber 5, carbs 25, protein 8

Amazing Potato Cakes

Opt for these today! They are so tasty!

Preparation time: 10 minutes
Cooking time: 10 minutes
Servings: 4

Ingredients:

- ¼ cup whole wheat flour
- A pinch of salt
- 1 teaspoon onion, minced
- 4 cups sweet potato, peeled and grated
- A pinch of nutmeg, ground
- Black pepper to the taste
- 1 egg, whisked
- Cooking spray

Directions:

In a bowl, mix sweet potato with flour, onion, salt, pepper, nutmeg and egg and stir well. Spray a skillet with some cooking spray and heat it up over medium high heat. Shape cakes out of the mixture from the bowl, add them to pan, cook for 4 minutes on each side and transfer them to paper towels. Drain excess grease, divide cakes between plates and serve them in the morning if you are on a dash diet. Enjoy!

Nutrition: calories 256, fat 4, fiber 5, carbs 29, protein 4

Breakfast Orange Delight

This is so delicious and healthy at the same time! Try this smoothie for a dash diet breakfast!

Preparation time: 5 minutes
Cooking time: 0 minutes
Servings: 2

Ingredients:
- 1 cup low fat milk
- 1 cup orange juice
- 6 ounces low-fat yogurt
- 20 ounces strawberries, frozen and thawed

Directions:

In your blender mix orange juice with milk, yogurt and strawberries and whisk well. Divide into 2 glasses and serve. Enjoy!

Nutrition: calories 100, fat 3, fiber 4, carbs 11, protein 1

Delicious Omelet

Have you ever tried a dash diet omelet? Then it's time to get to work!

Preparation time: 10 minutes
Cooking time: 5 minutes
Servings: 4

Ingredients:
- 8 eggs, whisked
- Cooking spray
- Salt and black pepper to the taste
- 2 tablespoons chives, chopped
- A pinch of cayenne pepper
- 2 ounces cheddar cheese, grated
- 2 cups spinach, torn

For the red pepper relish:
- 2 tablespoons green onion, chopped
- 2/3 cup red pepper, chopped
- 1 tablespoon vinegar

Directions:

In a bowl, mix eggs with salt, pepper, cayenne and chives and stir well. Heat up a pan over medium high heat, spray it with cooking spray, add eggs, spread into the pan, stir and cook for 1 minute. Add cheese and the spinach and fold your omelet. Continue cooking until cheese melts and divide it into plates. In a bowl, mix red pepper with green onions, black pepper to the taste and the vinegar and stir well. Top your omelet with the relish and serve. Enjoy!

Nutrition: calories 200, fat 4, fiber 5, carbs 13, protein 5

Wonderful Breakfast Bowls

You need to taste this right away!

Preparation time: 10 minutes
Cooking time: 10 minutes
Servings: 4

Ingredients:
- 2 apples, peeled, cored and roughly chopped
- 1 tablespoon butter
- ½ teaspoon ginger, grated
- 1 tablespoon brown sugar
- A pinch of cinnamon, ground
- 6 ounces fat free yogurt
- 4 teaspoons honey
- 1 teaspoon lemon zest, grated
- ¼ cup low fat granola

Directions:
Heat up a pan with the butter over medium heat, add apples, stir and cook them for 5 minutes. Reduce temperature, add ginger, cinnamon and sugar, stir and cook for 5 minutes more. Take off heat, leave apples aside to cool down and divide them into bowls. Add lemon zest, yogurt and yogurt and stir gently. Drizzle honey, sprinkle granola at the end and serve. Enjoy!

Nutrition: calories 200, fat 3, fiber 5, carbs 9, protein 7

Breakfast Zucchini Muffins

These muffins are simply delicious!

Preparation time: 10 minutes
Cooking time: 20 minutes
Servings: 4

Ingredients:
- 1 tablespoon baking powder
- 2 cups flour
- ½ cup palm sugar
- 2 teaspoons lemon rind, grated
- A pinch of salt
- 1 cup zucchini, grated
- ¼ teaspoons nutmeg, ground
- 1 egg
- Cooking spray
- 3 tablespoons vegetable oil
- ¾ cup skim milk

Directions:
In a bowl, mix flour with sugar, baking powder, lemon rind, salt and nutmeg and stir well. In another bowl, mix zucchini with milk, egg and oil and stir well. Spray a muffin tray with cooking spray, divide zucchini mix into the tray, introduce in the oven at 400 degrees F and bake for 20 minutes. Leave muffins to cool down, divide them between plates and serve. Enjoy!

Nutrition: calories 160, fat 3, fiber 2, carbs 7, protein 2

Special Breakfast Crunch

This is savory and easy to make!

Preparation time: 10 minutes
Cooking time: 0 minutes
Servings: 6

Ingredients:
- 4 cups mixed orange, apple, grapes and pineapple pieces
- 2 tablespoons honey
- ½ cup whole wheat and barley cereals
- 12 ounces low fat vanilla yogurt
- ¼ cup coconut, toasted and shredded

Directions:
Divide mixed fruits in 6 breakfast bowl, add yogurt and stir gently. Sprinkle cereals and toasted coconut on top and serve right away. Enjoy!

Nutrition: calories 130, fat 3, fiber 3, carbs 6, protein 3

Tasty Stuffed Peaches

Try these for a dash diet breakfast! You won't regret it!

Preparation time: 10 minutes
Cooking time: 40 minutes
Servings: 4

Ingredients:
- ½ cup dried fruits
- ¼ cup almonds, toasted
- 4 peaches, pitted and halved
- 2 tablespoons graham crackers, crumbled
- ¼ teaspoon allspice, ground
- 2 tablespoons brown sugar
- ½ cup fat free vanilla yogurt
- 12 ounces canned peach nectar

Directions:
Scoop each peach half, chop pulp and put into a bowl. Add dried fruits to this bowl and mix. Also add almonds, crackers, sugar and allspice and stir everything. Stuff each peach with this mix, place them on a baking sheet, add nectar all over, introduce in the oven at 350 degrees F and bake for 40 minutes. Divide peaches on plates, drizzle pan juices, top with yogurt and serve. Enjoy!

Nutrition: calories 230, fat 1, fiber 3, carbs 7, protein 5

Delicious Breakfast Parfait

This dash diet parfait is exceptional!

Preparation time: 10 minutes
Cooking time: 0 minutes
Servings: 6

Ingredients:

- 3 tablespoons honey
- 1 cup fat free yogurt
- 2 and ¼ teaspoons vanilla extract
- 1 and ½ cups papaya, chopped
- 6 tablespoons granola
- 1 and ½ cups pineapple, cut into medium pieces
- 1 and ½ cups strawberries, cut into medium pieces

Directions:

In a bowl, mix honey with yogurt and vanilla extract and stir. Divide papaya, strawberries and pineapple pieces into tall glasses, add yogurt mixture and stir gently. Top with granola and serve. Enjoy!

Nutrition: calories 140, fat 3, fiber 3, carbs 7, protein 3

Amazing Breakfast Smoothie

This is perfect for breakfast today!

Preparation time: 10 minutes
Cooking time: 0 minutes
Servings: 4

Ingredients:

- 1 cup cantaloupe, chopped
- 1 and ½ cups watermelon, seeded and chopped
- ¼ cup orange juice
- ½ cup low fat yogurt
- Watermelon wedges for serving

Directions:

In your blender, mix yogurt with watermelon and cantaloupe and pulse. Add orange juice, blend again, divide into glasses and serve with watermelon wedges on top. Enjoy!

Nutrition: calories 140, fat 1, fiber 3, carbs 7, protein 3

Breakfast Fruit Soup

Have you ever considered trying such a breakfast recipe?

Preparation time: 1 hour and 10 minutes
Cooking time: 0 minutes
Servings: 4

Ingredients:

- 2 cups cantaloupe, cut into medium pieces
- 1 and ½ cups canned peach nectar
- 6 ounces peach, pitted, peeled and cut into medium pieces
- 2 tablespoons lemon juice
- 1 cup raspberries
- A few mint leaves, torn

Directions:

In your blender, mix cantaloupe with peach nectar, peach and lemon juice and pulse well. Transfer to a bowl, cover and keep in the fridge fro 1 hour. Divide this into bowl, top with raspberries and mint leaves and serve, Enjoy!

Nutrition: calories 120, fat 1, fiber 1, carbs 0, protein 3

Tasty Summer Compote

If you are following a dash diet, then you should really try this breakfast idea as soon as possible!

Preparation time: 10 minutes
Cooking time: 20 minutes
Servings: 4

Ingredients:

- 2 tablespoons white wine vinegar
- 2 cups blueberries
- ½ cup palm sugar
- 2 tablespoons lemon juice
- ½ teaspoon lemon zest, grated
- 2 peaches, pitted, peeled and cut into wedges
- 1 and ½ cups raspberries
- 1 and ½ cups blackberries

Directions:

In a small pot, mix blueberries with sugar, vinegar, lemon juice and lemon zest, stir, bring to a boil over medium heat, simmer for 20 minutes, take off heat and leave aside to cool down. Divide this into 4 bowls, top with raspberries, blackberries and peach wedges and serve right away. Enjoy!

Nutrition: calories 120, fat 1, fiber 1, carbs 0, protein 4

Delicious French Toast

This is more than you expect!

Preparation time: 10 minutes
Cooking time: 10 minutes
Servings: 8

Ingredients:

- Cooking spray
- 8 French toast slices
- ½ cup fat free cream cheese
- 2 tablespoons strawberries, finely chopped
- 2 egg whites
- ¾ cup fat free milk
- 1 egg, whisked
- A pinch apple pie spice
- ½ teaspoon vanilla extract
- ½ cup strawberry spreadable fruit

Directions:

In a bowl, mix 2 tablespoons strawberries with cream cheese and stir well.
Create a pocket horizontally in each French toast slice and stuff them with cream cheese mix. In a bowl, mix egg white with milk, egg, apple spice and vanilla and stir well. Dip each bread slice in eggs mix. Heat up a pan with cooking spray over medium high heat, add bread slices, cook them for 2 minutes, flip and cook for 2 minutes more. Heat up spreadable fruit in a small pan over medium heat and spread over French toast. Divide between plates and serve. Enjoy!

Nutrition: calories 230, fat 6, fiber 3, carbs 7, protein 3

Breakfast Banana Smoothie

This is very healthy and easy to make!

Preparation time: 5 minutes
Cooking time: 0 minutes
Servings: 3

Ingredients:

- 10 strawberries, halved
- ½ teaspoon vanilla extract
- 1 and ½ cups vanilla soy milk
- 1 and ½ tablespoons honey
- 1 cup fat free whipped topping
- 1 banana, peeled and sliced

Directions:

In your blender, mix strawberries with vanilla, soy milk, banana and honey and pulse well.
Divide into glasses, top with whipped topping and serve. Enjoy!

Nutrition: calories 150, fat 3, fiber 2, carbs 7, protein 4

Breakfast Oatmeal

This dash diet oatmeal is just what you need today!

Preparation time: 10 minutes
Cooking time: 5 minutes
Servings: 4

Ingredients:

- 4 cups water
- 3 cups rolled oats
- 3 cups whole grain cereal flakes
- 1 cup apples, dried and chopped
- 1 cup dates, dried and chopped
- 1 cup walnuts, chopped
- 2 tablespoons cinnamon, ground
- 1 cup coconut sugar
- 1 teaspoon cloves, ground
- 1 tablespoon ginger, ground
- 1 teaspoon turmeric ground

Directions:

Put the water into a pot and bring to a boil over medium high heat. Divide oats, cereal flakes, apples, walnuts, cinnamon, sugar, ginger, cloves and turmeric into bowls and stir them. Add boiling water over them, cover bowls and leave them aside for 10 minutes. Serve right away. Enjoy!

Nutrition: calories 150, fat 3, fiber 6, carbs 10, protein 3

Scrambled Eggs

Serve for breakfast today!

Preparation time: 10 minutes
Cooking time: 10 minutes
Servings: 4

Ingredients:

- 3 eggs
- ¼ cup green bell pepper, chopped
- ¾ cup tomato, chopped
- Cooking spray
- ¼ cup green onions, chopped
- 1 and ½ cups eggs replacement
- ¼ cup fat free milk
- A pinch of salt and black pepper
- A splash of hot pepper

Directions:

Heat up a pan with some cooking spray over medium high heat, add bell pepper, tomato and onions, stir, cook for 5 minutes and transfer to a bowl. In another bowl, mix eggs with egg replacement, milk, salt, pepper and hot sauce and whisk really well. Heat up the same pan again over medium high heat, add eggs mix, cook them until they are done stirring often. Divide scrambled eggs on plates, top with sautéed veggies and serve. Enjoy!

Nutrition: calories 140, fat 2, fiber 3, carbs 5, protein 5

Special Breakfast Casserole

This is very healthy and it follows the dash diet principles!

Preparation time: 10 minutes
Cooking time: 45 minutes
Servings: 8

Ingredients:

- ¾ cup canned enchilada sauce
- 15 ounces canned black beans, drained
- 8 ounces canned green chili peppers, chopped
- A splash of hot pepper sauce
- ½ cup green onions, chopped
- Cooking spray
- 1 cup cheddar cheese, grated
- 2 garlic cloves, minced
- 3 egg whites
- 2 tablespoons flour
- 3 egg yolks
- A pinch of salt
- ½ cup fat free milk
- 1 tablespoon cilantro, chopped

Directions:

Grease a baking dish with cooking spray and add beans, chili peppers, enchilada sauce, green onions, pepper sauce, salt, garlic and cheese. In a bowl, beat egg whites with a mixer. In a separate bowl, mix egg yolks with salt and flour and whisk well. Add egg whites, milk and cilantro and whisk well again. Pour this over beans mix, spread well, introduce in the oven at 325 degrees F and bake for 45 minutes. Leave casserole to cool down, divide between plates and serve for breakfast. Enjoy!

Nutrition: calories 240, fat 4, fiber 3, carbs 6, protein 6

Breakfast Frittata

This is one breakfast idea worth trying!

Preparation time: 10 minutes
Cooking time: 10 minutes
Servings: 4

Ingredients:

- 4 ounces shrimp, peeled, deveined and cut into halves horizontally
- 2 cups egg product
- 4 ounces canned artichokes, drained and chopped
- ¼ cup fat free milk
- A pinch of black pepper
- A pinch of garlic powder
- ¼ cup green onions, chopped
- Cooking spray
- 3 tablespoons cheddar cheese, grated
- 8 cherry tomatoes, halved
- 1 tablespoon parsley, chopped

Directions:

In a bowl, mix egg product with milk, black pepper, garlic powder and green onions and stir well. Heat up a pan with the cooking spray over medium high heat, add shrimp, stir and cook for 3 minutes. Add eggs mix, spread, reduce heat to medium-low, cook until the mix is almost done and take off heat. Sprinkle artichokes, cheddar cheese, tomatoes and parsley on top, cover pan and leave aside for 4 minutes. Divide frittata between plates and serve. Enjoy!

Nutrition: calories 200, fat 2, fiber 3, carbs 5, protein 4

Breakfast Quinoa Pancakes

These are extremely tasty and easy to make!

Preparation time: 10 minutes
Cooking time: 30 minutes
Servings: 4

Ingredients:

- 1 and ½ cups water
- 2 garlic cloves, minced
- ¾ cup quinoa
- 2 egg whites
- A pinch of salt
- ½ cup parmesan, grated
- Black pepper to the taste
- ½ teaspoon basil, dried
- 6 cups baby spinach leaves
- 1 cups salsa
- 4 teaspoons olive oil

Directions:

Put the water in a pan and bring to a boil over medium high heat. Add quinoa, salt and the garlic, stir, cover, simmer for 10 minutes, uncover pan, cook for 2 minutes more, take off heat, drain, transfer to a bowl, fluff with a fork and cool down. Add parmesan, basil, black pepper and egg whites and whisk everything well. Heat up a pan with half of the oil over medium heat, make 2 pancakes out of the quinoa mix, place them in the pan, cook for 2 minutes on each side and transfer them to a lined baking sheet. Add the rest of the oil to the pan and also heat up over medium high heat. Make 2 more quinoa pancakes, cook them for 2 minutes on each side and also transfer them to the baking sheet. Introduce pancakes in the oven at 350 degrees F for 5 minutes and divide them between plates. Serve in the morning with salsa on top. Enjoy!

Nutrition: calories 170, fat 4, fiber 4, carbs 7, protein 3

Amazing Tofu Scramble

It's time for a delicious tofu scramble!

Preparation time: 10 minutes
Cooking time: 10 minutes
Servings: 4

Ingredients:

- 18 ounces package firm tofu, drained well, pat dried and crumbled
- 2 poblano chili peppers, chopped
- 1 tablespoon olive oil
- 2 garlic cloves, minced
- ½ cup onion, chopped
- 1 teaspoon chili powder
- ½ teaspoon oregano, dried
- ½ teaspoon cumin, ground
- A pinch of sea salt
- 2 tomatoes, peeled and chopped
- 1 tablespoon lime juice
- 1 tablespoon cilantro, chopped

Directions:

Heat up a pan with the oil over medium high heat, add chili peppers, garlic and onion, stir and cook for 4 minutes. Add salt, chili powder, oregano and cumin, stir and cook for 1 minute more. Add tofu, stir, reduce heat and cook for 5 minutes more. Add tomatoes, lime juice and cilantro, stir well again, divide between plates and serve. Enjoy!

Nutrition: calories 150, fat 3, fiber 2, carbs 5, protein 3

Delicious Squash and Apples

This is a really interesting and delicious dash diet side dish!

Preparation time: 10 minutes
Cooking time: 15 minutes
Servings: 2

Ingredients:

- 1 big apple, cored, peeled and cut into wedges
- 1 acorn squash, halved
- 2 tablespoons brown sugar
- 2 teaspoons fat free margarine

Directions:

In a bowl, mix apple pieces with sugar and stir well. Pierce acorn squash pieces a few times, arrange on a lined baking sheet, introduce in the oven at 400 degrees F for 10 minutes, leave it aside to cool down, scrape seeds and fill each piece with the apple mix. Introduce in the oven again at 400 degrees F and bake for 6 minutes more. Divide margarine when squash halves are still hot, divide between plates and serve as a side for a pork main dish. Enjoy!

Nutrition: calories 200, fat 5, fiber 6, carbs 40, protein 3

Stuffed Artichokes

This is a really great side dish if you are on a Dash diet!

Preparation time: 10 minutes
Cooking time: 55 minutes
Servings: 8

Ingredients:

- 4 artichokes, trimmed and insides scooped out
- 2 cups whole wheat breadcrumbs
- 1 tablespoon olive oil
- Juice of 1 lemon
- 3 garlic cloves, minced
- 1/3 cup parmesan, grated
- 1 tablespoon lemon zest, grated
- 2 tablespoons parsley, chopped
- Black pepper to the taste
- 1 cup vegetable stock
- 2 tablespoons vegetable stock
- 1 tablespoon shallot, minced
- 1 cup white wine
- 1 teaspoon oregano, chopped

Directions:

In a bowl, mix breadcrumbs with the oil, stir well, spread on a lined baking sheet, introduce in the oven at 400 degrees F, toast for 10 minutes and leave them aside to cool down. Rub artichokes with the lemon juice and place them on a working surface. In a bowl, mix cold bread crumbs with garlic, parsley, parmesan, lemon zest, black pepper and 2 tablespoons vegetable stock, stir really well and stuff each artichoke with this mix Put the rest of the stock, wine, oregano and shallot into a pot, bring to a boil over medium heat, stir, add artichokes, cover pot and simmer for 45 minutes. Leave stuffed artichokes to cool down, cut each into quarters, arrange on plates and serve. Enjoy!

Nutrition: calories 200, fat 4, fiber 4, carbs 20, protein 6

Amazing Asparagus Dish

This dash diet side dish is full of nutrients and vitamins and it tastes great!

Preparation time: 10 minutes
Cooking time: 5 minutes
Servings: 4

Ingredients:

- 1 pound asparagus, trimmed and ends removed
- 1 tablespoon parsley, chopped
- 1 garlic clove, minced
- ¼ teaspoon lemon zest, grated
- 1 tablespoon hazelnuts, toasted
- 2 teaspoons lemon juice
- 1 teaspoon lemon zest, grated
- A pinch of sea salt

Directions:

Put some water in a pot, add a steamer basket inside, bring to a boil over medium heat, add asparagus, boil for 5 minutes, discard water and transfer asparagus to a bowl filled with ice water. Drain asparagus again and transfer it to a bowl. Add salt, garlic, parsley, lemon zest, lemon juice, hazelnuts and oil and stir everything. Divide between plates and serve. Enjoy!

Nutrition: calories 60, fat 3, fiber 2, carbs 6, protein 4

Minted Carrots

This is really flavored and delicious!

Preparation time: 10 minutes
Cooking time: 15 minutes
Servings: 6

Ingredients:

- 6 cups water
- ¼ cup apple juice
- 1 pound baby carrots
- 1 tablespoon cornstarch
- A pinch of cinnamon
- ½ tablespoon mint, chopped

Directions:

Put the water in a pot, bring to a boil over medium heat, add carrots, cook for 10 minutes, drain and transfer them to a bowl. Heat up a small pan with the apple juice over medium heat, add cornstarch, mint and cinnamon, stir, cook for 4-5 minutes and take off heat. Drizzle this over carrots, divide them between plates and serve as a side if you are on a dash diet. Enjoy!

Nutrition: calories 50, fat 2, fiber 2, carbs 8, protein 1

Black Bean Relish

This is just unbelievable!

Preparation time: 40 minutes
Cooking time: 0 minutes
Servings: 8

Ingredients:

- 4 tomatoes, chopped
- 1 cup corn kernels
- 16 ounces canned black beans, drained
- 2 garlic cloves, minced
- ½ cup parsley, chopped
- 1 small red onion, chopped
- 1 red bell pepper, chopped
- Juice of 1 lemon
- 2 tablespoons stevia

Directions:

In a large bowl, mix tomatoes with corn, black beans, garlic, parsley, lemon juice, bell pepper, onion and stevia and stir well. Keep this in the fridge for about 30 minutes before serving as a side. Enjoy!

Nutrition: calories 100, fat 1, fiber 5, carbs 20, protein 7

Simple Black Bean Cakes

We know for sure that this is a really special and delicious dash diet side! You should try it for sure!

Preparation time: 1 hour and 10 minutes
Cooking time: 1 hour and 10 minutes
Servings: 6

Ingredients:

- 4 cups water
- 2 cups black beans, soaked overnight and drained
- Salt and black pepper to the taste
- 8 garlic cloves, minced
- ½ cup cilantro, chopped
- 2 tablespoons olive oil

Directions:

Put the water in a pot, add beans, bring to a boil over medium heat, reduce temperature, cover pot partially and cook beans for 1 hour. Drain black beans, transfer them to a bowl and mash using a potato masher. Add salt, pepper, cilantro and garlic and stir well. Shape 8 patties out of this mix, place them all on a lined baking sheet and keep in the fridge for 1 hour. Heat up a pan with the oil over medium high heat, add black beans patties, cook them for 3 minutes, flip, cook for another 3 minutes and divide them between plates. Serve as a side dish right away! Enjoy!

Nutrition: calories 200, fat 4, fiber 6, carbs 40, protein 10

Delicious Celery Root

We thought you could use more delicious dash diet sides! Therefore, here's another one!

Preparation time: 10 minutes
Cooking time: 15 minutes
Servings: 6

Ingredients:

- 1 celery root, chopped
- 1 cup veggie stock
- 1 teaspoon mustard
- ¼ cup sour cream
- Salt and black pepper to the taste
- 2 teaspoons thyme, chopped

Directions:

Put the stock in a pot and bring to a boil over medium high heat. Add celery, stir, bring to a simmer, cover and cook over medium heat for 10 minutes. Transfer celery pieces to a bowl and leave aside for now. Bring the liquid from the pot to a boil again over medium heat, cook for 5 minutes and take off heat again. Add salt, pepper, mustard and sour cream and stir well. Return celery to pot, also add thyme, stir, divide between plates and serve as a side. Enjoy!

Nutrition: calories 70, fat 2, fiber 1, carbs 6, protein 2

Amazing Kale and Cherry Tomatoes

This is a really delicious combination you can try today!

Preparation time: 10 minutes
Cooking time: 15 minutes
Servings: 6

Ingredients:

- 1 pound kale, chopped
- 2 teaspoons olive oil
- 4 garlic cloves, minced
- ½ cup veggie stock
- 1 tablespoons lemon juice
- 1 cup cherry tomatoes, halved
- Black pepper to the taste

Directions:

Heat up a pan with the oil over medium heat, add garlic, stir and cook for 2 minutes. Add kale and stock, stir, cover and cook for 5 minutes more. Add tomatoes, stir and cook for 7 minutes more. Take this off heat, add black pepper and lemon juice, stir, divide between plates and serve right away as a side dish. Enjoy!

Nutrition: calories 80, fat 2, fiber 3, carbs 8, protein 5

Tasty Broccoli

This is so tasty and delicious! It will surprise you!

Preparation time: 10 minutes
Cooking time: 4 minutes
Servings: 4

Ingredients:

- 1 teaspoon olive oil
- 4 cups broccoli florets
- 1 teaspoon lemon zest, grated
- 1 tablespoon garlic, minced
- A pinch of salt
- Black pepper to the taste
- 1 cup water

Directions:

Put the water in a pot, bring to a boil over medium heat, add broccoli, cook for 3 minutes, drain and put into a bowl. Heat up a pan with the oil over medium high heat, add garlic, stir and cook for 1 minute. Add broccoli, salt, pepper and lemon zest, stir, take off heat, divide between plates and serve right away. Enjoy!

Nutrition: calories 60, fat 1, fiber 3, carbs 7, protein 3

Special Brown Rice Pilaf

This is one of our favorite dash diet sides!

Preparation time: 10 minutes
Cooking time: 35 minutes
Servings: 6

Ingredients:

- 3 cups water
- 1 cup brown rice
- 1 tablespoon olive oil
- 1 teaspoon bouillon granules
- A pinch of nutmeg, ground
- ½ pound mushrooms, sliced
- 1 yellow onion, chopped
- ½ pound asparagus tips
- 2 tablespoons Swiss cheese, grated
- ½ cup parsley, chopped

Directions:

Heat up a pan with the oil over medium heat, add rice, toast it for a few minutes and mix with the water. Add bouillon, onions, nutmeg and mushrooms, stir, bring to a boil, cover, reduce heat and simmer for 30 minutes. Add asparagus, stir and cook for 5 minutes more. Take off heat, divide between plates and serve as a side dish with cheese and parsley on top. Enjoy!

Nutrition: calories 180, fat 1, fiber 2, carbs 27, protein 7

Cheese Zucchinis

Get your ingredients and make this side dish today!

Preparation time: 10 minutes
Cooking time: 38 minutes
Servings: 2

Ingredients:

- 1 zucchini, sliced
- ½ teaspoon garlic powder
- 1 teaspoon olive oil
- 1/8 teaspoon onion powder
- 2 tablespoons parmesan, grated

Directions:

Pat dry zucchini slices and arrange them all on a lined baking sheet. Season with onion and garlic powder, drizzle the oil, toss well, introduce in the oven at 375 degrees F and bake for 35 minutes. Sprinkle parmesan on top and bake for 3 minutes more. Divide between plates and serve. Enjoy!

Nutrition: calories 70, fat 4, fiber 1, carbs 4, protein 3

Classic Baked Beans

This side dish is perfect for a family meal!

Preparation time: 10 minutes
Cooking time: 6 hours
Servings: 12

Ingredients:

- 3 bacon strips, chopped
- ½ cup molasses
- 1 yellow onion, chopped
- 1 and ½ tablespoons dry mustard
- A pinch of salt
- 2 bay leaves
- 4 water cups
- 2 cups navy beans, soaked overnight and drained

Directions:

In a big pot, mix beans with water, bay leaves and a pinch of salt, stir, bring to a boil over medium high heat, cover, reduce temperature and simmer for 1 hour. Drain beans, return them to the pot and mix with bacon, molasses, mustard and onion. Stir, cover pot and bake in the oven at 350 degrees F and bake for 5 hours. Divide baked beans between plates and serve them as a dash diet side! Enjoy!

Nutrition: calories 170, fat 3, fiber 8, carbs 20, protein 7

Delicious Corn Pudding

This is another tasty and classic dash diet side dish you need to try soon!

Preparation time: 10 minutes
Cooking time: 15 minutes
Servings: 8

Ingredients:

- 3 cups skim milk
- 3 cups water
- ¼ cup maple syrup
- 2 cups cornmeal
- A pinch of nutmeg, ground
- ¼ teaspoon cinnamon, ground
- A pinch of cloves, ground
- ½ cup raisins
- A pinch of ginger ground

Directions:

Put the milk and water in a pot, stir and bring to a boil over medium high heat. Add cornmeal, bring to a boil again, cover, reduce temperature and cook for 10 minutes stirring often. Take off heat, add raisins, maple syrup, nutmeg, cinnamon, cloves and ginger, stir, cover again and leave aside for 10 minutes. Divide between plates and serve as a side. Enjoy!

Nutrition: calories 200, fat 1, fiber 2, carbs 24, protein 7

Incredible Swiss Chard

This is such a delightful side dish!

Preparation time: 10 minutes
Cooking time: 5 minutes
Servings: 6

Ingredients:
- 1 and ½ tablespoons flour
- 2 tablespoons olive oil
- 1 and ¼ cups soy milk
- 2 pound Swiss chard, cut into strips
- 3 garlic cloves, minced
- A pinch of salt and black pepper
- 1 tablespoon parmesan, grated

Directions:

Heat up a pan with the oil over medium high heat, add flour and stir until you obtain a paste. Add garlic, stir and cook for 1 minute more. Add soy milk, stir and cook for 1 minute more. Add chard, stir, cover and cook for 2 minutes. Add salt, pepper and parmesan, stir a bit, divide between plates and serve. Enjoy!

Nutrition: calories 101, fat 4, fiber 3, carbs 7, protein 5

Amazing and Delicious Eggplant

It's delicious, spicy and flavored!

Preparation time: 10 minutes
Cooking time: 15 minutes
Servings: 4

Ingredients:
- 1 eggplant, sliced
- ½ teaspoon cumin, ground
- 1 teaspoon mustard seed
- ½ teaspoon coriander, ground
- ½ teaspoon curry powder
- A pinch of nutmeg, ground
- A pinch of ginger, ground
- A pinch of cloves, ground
- 2 cups cherry tomatoes, halved
- ½ yellow onion, chopped
- 1 tablespoon olive oil
- 1 garlic clove, minced
- 1 tablespoon molasses
- 1 teaspoon red wine vinegar
- A pinch of salt
- Black pepper to the taste
- 1 tablespoon cilantro, chopped

Directions:

Place eggplant slices into a pan, introduce in your preheated broiler and brown them for 5 minutes on each side. In a bowl, mix mustard seeds with cumin, coriander, curry , ginger, nutmeg and cloves and stir. Heat up a pan with the oil over medium high heat, add spices and toast them for 30 seconds. Add onion, stir and sauté for 4 minutes. Add garlic, molasses, tomatoes and vinegar, stir and cook for 4 minutes more. Add salt, pepper and eggplant slices. Leave them in the pan for a few minutes, then divide between plates and serve as a side. Enjoy!

Nutrition: calories 140, fat 4, fiber 5, carbs 20, protein 4

Asian Side Salad

This great Asian inspired salad is perfect for you today!

Preparation time: 10 minutes
Cooking time: 0 minutes
Servings: 4

Ingredients:
- 1 and ½ cups carrots, grated
- 1 and ½ cups snow peas
- 1 and ½ cups spinach, cut into thin strips
- 1 and ½ cups bok choy, cut into thin strips
- ½ cups yellow onion, chopped
- 2 teaspoons sesame oil
- 2 teaspoons low sodium soy sauce
- 1 tablespoon cilantro, chopped
- 1 tablespoon garlic, minced
- 1 cup red cabbage, shredded
- 1 and ½ tablespoons cashews, chopped
- ½ cup red bell pepper, chopped

Directions:

In a large bowl, mix carrots with snow peas, spinach, bok choy, onion, cilantro, garlic, cabbage, cashews and bell pepper and stir. Add sesame oil and soy sauce, toss to coat well and serve as a side for a shrimp based dish. Enjoy!

Nutrition: calories 100, fat 4, fiber 3, carbs 10, protein 3

Glazed Sweet Potatoes

This dash diet side dish is more than you could expect!

Preparation time: 10 minutes
Cooking time: 1 hour
Servings: 8

Ingredients:
- 2 tablespoons brown sugar
- ¼ cup water
- 1 tablespoon olive oil
- 2 tablespoons honey
- 4 sweet potatoes, peeled and cut into wedges
- Black pepper to the taste
- A pinch of rosemary, dried

Directions:

Coat a baking dish with some oil and arrange potato wedges inside. In a bowl, mix water with oil, sugar and honey and whisk well. Pour this over potatoes, toss to coat, cover the dish, introduce in the oven at 350 degrees F and bake for 45 minutes. Uncover baking dish and cook glazed potatoes for 15 minutes more. Sprinkle black pepper and rosemary on top, divide potatoes between plates and serve as a side dish. Enjoy!

Nutrition: calories 150, fat 3, fiber 4, carbs 32, protein 2

Amazing Lima Beans and Tomatoes

The combination is really good!

Preparation time: 10 minutes
Cooking time: 20 minutes
Servings: 6

Ingredients:

- 2 tablespoons olive oil
- 1 tomato, chopped
- 4 pounds lima beans
- 3 garlic cloves, minced
- 1 small yellow onion, chopped
- 1 bay leaf
- 1 and ½ teaspoon thyme, chopped
- A pinch of salt
- 1 cup veggie stock
- 2 tablespoons parsley, chopped

Directions:

Put water in a pot, bring to a boil over medium heat, add beans, stir a bit, cook for 6 minutes, drain them and leave aside for now. Heat up a pan with half of the oil over medium heat, add garlic, onion, tomato, bay leaf, a pinch of salt and thyme, stir and sauté them for 5 minutes. Add stock, stir, bring to a boil, reduce heat to medium-low and mix with beans. Stir again and cook everything for 3 minutes. Discard bay leaf, divide beans mix between plates and serve as a side dish with the rest of the oil drizzled on top and with parsley sprinkled all over. Enjoy!

Nutrition: calories 179, fat 3, fiber 4, carbs 25, protein 6

Delicious Sautéed Corn

You will simply adore this great dash diet side dish!

Preparation time: 10 minutes
Cooking time: 12 minutes
Servings: 6

Ingredients:

- 2 ounces prosciutto, cut into strips
- 1 teaspoon olive oil
- 2 cups corn kernels
- 1 teaspoon garlic, minced
- 1 green bell pepper, chopped

Directions:

Heat up a pan with the oil over medium heat, add prosciutto pieces, stir and cook for 5 minutes. Add garlic, corn and bell pepper, stir and cook for 7 minutes more. Divide between plates and serve right away as a side dish. Enjoy!

Nutrition: calories 89, fat 2, fiber 2, carbs 10, protein 5

Spicy and Delicious Cabbage

This is a great and delicious dash diet side dish!

Preparation time: 10 minutes
Cooking time: 1 hour
Servings: 6

Ingredients:

- 1 apple, cored, peeled and chopped
- 2 yellow onions, chopped
- 10 cups red cabbage, shredded
- 1 cup prunes, pitted and chopped
- 1 teaspoon cinnamon, ground
- 1 garlic clove, minced
- 1 teaspoon cumin seeds
- ¼ teaspoon cloves, ground
- 2 tablespoons red wine vinegar
- 1 teaspoon coriander seeds
- ½ cup water
- A pinch of nutmeg

Directions:

In a pot, mix cabbage with onions, apple, prunes, garlic, cinnamon, cumin, cloves, vinegar, coriander, nutmeg and water, stir, bring to a simmer over medium heat and cook for 1 hour. Stir again, divide between plates and serve as a side dish. Enjoy!

Nutrition: calories 147, fat 1, fiber 5, carbs 34, protein 3

Dash Diet Snacks and Appetizers Recipes

Apple Slices and Tasty Dip

You can serve this dash diet snack on a casual gathering!

Preparation time: 10 minutes
Cooking time: 0 minutes
Servings: 4

Ingredients:

- 2 tablespoons brown sugar
- 8 ounces fat free cream cheese
- 2 tablespoons peanuts, chopped
- 4 medium apples, cored and sliced
- 1 and ½ teaspoons vanilla extract
- ½ cup orange juice

Directions:

In a bowl, mix cream cheese with sugar, vanilla and peanuts and whisk well. Arrange apple slices on a platter and drizzle orange juice over them. Serve with the cream cheese dip on the side. Enjoy!

Nutrition: calories 110, fat 1, fiber 2, carbs 10, protein 4

Tasty Artichoke Dip

This goes perfectly with some carrot or celery sticks!

Preparation time: 10 minutes
Cooking time: 30 minutes
Servings: 8

Ingredients:

- 4 cups spinach, chopped
- 2 cups artichoke hearts
- Black pepper to the taste
- 1 teaspoon thyme, chopped
- 2 garlic cloves, minced
- 1 cup white beans, already cooked
- 1 tablespoon parsley, chopped
- 2 tablespoons low fat parmesan, grated
- ½ cup low fat sour cream

Directions:

In a baking dish, mix artichokes with spinach, black pepper, thyme, garlic, beans, parsley, parmesan and sour cream, stir well, introduce in the oven at 350 degrees F and bake for 30 minutes. Mash using a potato masher, divide into bowls and serve with veggie sticks. Enjoy!

Nutrition: calories 100, fat 2, fiber 6, carbs 13, protein 5

Tasty Avocado Dip

This delicious avocado dip is perfect!

Preparation time: 10 minutes
Cooking time: 0 minutes
Servings: 4

Ingredients:

- 2 teaspoons onion, chopped
- 1 avocado, peeled, pitted and mashed with a fork
- ½ cup fat free sour cream
- A splash of hot sauce

Directions:

In a bowl, mix sour cream with onion, avocado and hot sauce, whisk well and serve right away. Enjoy!

Nutrition: calories 89, fat 1, fiber 2, carbs 7, protein 2

Simple Eggplant Dip

This is very flavored and it can be served both warm and cold!

Preparation time: 10 minutes
Cooking time: 36 minutes
Servings: 4

Ingredients:

- 2 eggplants, sliced lengthwise
- 1 garlic head, top cut off
- 1 red bell pepper, halved
- 1 tablespoon olive oil
- Black pepper to the taste
- 1 tablespoon basil, chopped
- 4 tablespoons lemon juice
- Cooking spray

Directions:

Spray your grill with some cooking spray and heat it up over medium high heat. Wrap garlic head in some tin foil, place on grill and roast for 30 minutes. Leave garlic to cool down and then squeeze it into a bowl. Place eggplant slices and bell pepper halves on preheat grill, roast them for 3 minutes on each side and transfer them to a cutting board. Once veggies are cold, transfer them to your food processor. Add garlic, oil, black pepper, basil and lemon juice and blend everything well. Transfer to a bowl and serve with warm pita bread on the side. Enjoy!

Nutrition: calories 150, fat 2, fiber 3, carbs 20, protein 4

Delicious Stuffed Mushrooms

These look incredible and they taste delicious! Serve them as a dash diet appetizer!

Preparation time: 10 minutes
Cooking time: 15 minutes
Servings: 20

Ingredients:

- 20 mushrooms, stems removed
- ¼ cup low fat butter, melted
- 1 and ½ cups panko breadcrumbs
- 2 tablespoons parsley, chopped
- 2 tablespoons pumpkin seeds
- 2 cups basil, chopped
- ¼ cup low fat parmesan, grated
- 1 tablespoon garlic, minced
- 2 teaspoons lemon juice
- 1 tablespoon olive oil
- A pinch of sea salt

Directions:

In a bowl, mix butter with panko and parsley, stir well and leave aside. In your blender, mix basil with pumpkin seeds, oil, parmesan, garlic, a pinch of salt and lemon juice and pulse really well. Arrange mushrooms on a lined baking sheet, divide basil mix in each and top with panko mixture. Introduce them in the oven at 350 degrees F and bake for 15 minutes. Arrange mushrooms on platters and serve as a dash diet appetizer! Enjoy!

Nutrition: calories 60, fat 1, fiber 0, carbs 4, protein 2

Spicy Shrimp

Shrimp are the best! Try this appetizer soon!

Preparation time: 10 minutes
Cooking time: 10 minutes
Servings: 4

Ingredients:

- 48 medium shrimp, pat dried, peeled and deveined
- 1 and ½ teaspoons water
- 2 tablespoons tomato paste
- ½ teaspoon olive oil
- ½ teaspoon chipotle chili powder
- ½ teaspoon oregano, chopped
- ½ teaspoon garlic, minced

Directions:

In a bowl, mix water with tomato paste, oil, chili powder, oregano and garlic and whisk really well. Add shrimp, toss to coat well and keep in the fridge for 10 minutes. Preheat your kitchen grill over medium high heat, arrange shrimp on it, grill them for 4 minutes on each side, transfer to a platter and serve them right away. Enjoy!

Nutrition: calories 90, fat 1, fiber 0.5, carbs 2, protein 10

Simple Coconut Shrimp

Here's another delicious dash diet appetizer idea! Try it for your next party!

Preparation time: 10 minutes
Cooking time: 15 minutes
Servings: 6

Ingredients:
- 12 big shrimp, peeled and deveined
- A pinch of sea salt
- ¼ cup panko bread crumbs
- ¼ cup coconut, shredded
- ½ cup coconut milk
- Cooking spray

Directions:
Spray a baking sheet with some cooking spray and leave it aside for now. In your food processor, mix panko with a pinch of salt and coconut, pulse well and transfer to a bowl. Put coconut milk in a second bowl. Dip shrimp in coconut milk, then in panko mix and arrange them on greased baking sheet. Introduce in the oven at 375 degrees F and bake for 15 minutes. Serve them warm. Enjoy!

Nutrition: calories 76, fat 2, fiber 0, carbs 3, protein 5

Wonderful Potato Skins

These potato skins are simply wonderful!

Preparation time: 10 minutes
Cooking time: 1 hour and 10 minutes
Servings: 2

Ingredients:
- Cooking spray
- 2 potatoes
- 1 tablespoon rosemary, chopped
- A pinch of black pepper

Directions:
Prick potatoes with a fork, place them on a baking sheet, introduce in the oven at 375 degrees F and bake for 1 hour. Cut potatoes into halves and scoop almost all the flesh. Spray potato skins with cooking spray, sprinkle black pepper and rosemary, introduce them in the oven again and bake for 10 minutes. Divide potato skins between plates and serve them right away. Enjoy!

Nutrition: calories 110, fat 0, fiber 4, carbs 20, protein 2

Great Tomato Crostini

This Italian style snack is so balanced and flavored!

Preparation time: 30 minutes
Cooking time: 0 minutes
Servings: 4

Ingredients:

- 2 teaspoons olive oil
- 4 tomatoes, chopped
- ¼ cup basil, chopped
- 1 garlic clove, minced
- 4 crusty Italian whole wheat bread slices, toasted
- Black pepper to the taste

Directions:

In a bowl, mix tomatoes with basil, garlic, oil and black pepper, stir, cover and keep in the fridge for 30 minutes. Divide this mix into toasted bread slices and serve right away. Enjoy!

Nutrition: calories 104, fat 1, fiber 1,carbs 10, protein 4

Simple Grilled Pineapple

You can even take this snack with you at the office!

Preparation time: 10 minutes
Cooking time: 10 minutes
Servings: 8

Ingredients:

- 1 tablespoon lime juice
- 2 tablespoons honey
- 1 tablespoon olive oil
- 1 teaspoon cinnamon, ground
- 1 pineapple, peeled and cut into medium pieces
- ¼ teaspoon cloves, ground
- 1 tablespoon dark rum
- 1 tablespoon lime zest, grated

Directions:

In a bowl, mix lime juice with honey, oil, cinnamon and cloves and whisk well. Brush pineapple pieces with this marinade, skewer them and place on preheated grill over medium high heat. Cook for 5 minutes on each side, basting with the marinade from time to time. Take them off heat, leave aside to cool down a bit, brush with rum, sprinkle lime zest and serve warm or cold. Enjoy!

Nutrition: calories 50, fat 1, fiber 1, carbs 10, protein 0.5

Delicious and Easy Hummus

This is so popular all over the world! Try it!

Preparation time: 10 minutes
Cooking time: 1 hour
Servings: 6

Ingredients:

- 2/3 cup chickpeas, soaked overnight and drained
- 2 garlic cloves
- 3 cups water
- 1 bay leaf
- 1 tablespoon olive oil
- A pinch of salt
- 2 tablespoons sherry vinegar
- ¾ cup green onions, chopped
- 1 teaspoon cumin, ground
- 3 tablespoons cilantro, chopped

Directions:

Put the water in a pot, add a pinch of salt and chickpeas and stir. Add garlic and bay leaf as well, stir, bring to a simmer, cover partially and cook for 1 hours. Discard bay leaf and liquid but reserve ½ cup. Transfer chickpeas to your food processor, add reserved liquid, green onions, vinegar, oil, garlic, cilantro and cumin and blend really well. Transfer to a bowl and serve. Enjoy!

Nutrition: calories 113, fat 1, fiber 3, carbs 10, protein 3

Fruit Kebabs

These are perfect for the summer!

Preparation time: 10 minutes
Cooking time: 0 minutes
Servings: 2

Ingredients:

- 1 teaspoon lime zest, grated
- 1 teaspoon lime juice
- 6 ounces sugar-free and low fat lemon yogurt
- 1 banana, peeled and cut in 4 medium wedges
- 4 strawberries
- 1 kiwi, peeled and cut into quarters
- 4 red grapes
- 4 pineapple pieces

Directions:

Thread banana pieces, strawberries, grapes, pineapple chunks and grapes on skewers alternating them and arrange on a platter. In a bowl, mix lemon yogurt with lime zest and lime juice, whisk well and keep in the fridge until you serve your fruit kebabs. Enjoy!

Nutrition: calories 145, fat 2, fiber 4, carbs 34, protein 4

Delicious Fruit Salsa

You've got to try this as soon as possible!

Preparation time: 2 hours and 10 minutes
Cooking time: 12 minutes
Servings: 10

Ingredients:
- 1 tablespoon brown sugar
- 8 whole wheat tortillas, cut into medium pieces
- ½ tablespoon cinnamon powder
- 3 cups mixed apples with oranges and grapes
- 1 tablespoon agave nectar
- 2 tablespoon sugar free jam
- 2 tablespoons orange juice

Directions:

In a bowl, combine mixed fruits with agave nectar, jam and orange juice, toss well, cover and keep in the fridge for 2 hours. Meanwhile, spread tortilla pieces on a lined baking sheet, sprinkle cinnamon powder and sugar all over them and bake in the oven at 350 degrees F for 12 minutes. Divide fruits salsa into bowls and serve with tortilla chips on the side. Enjoy!

Nutrition: calories 110, fat 2, fiber 2, carbs 20, protein 2

Pickled Asparagus

You will never forget this one snack!

Preparation time: 4 weeks
Cooking time: 0 minutes
Servings: 6

Ingredients:
- 3 cups asparagus spears, trimmed and cut in halves
- ¼ cup pearl onions
- ¼ cup apple cider vinegar
- 1 dill spring
- ¼ cup white wine vinegar
- 2 cloves
- 1 cup water
- 3 garlic cloves, sliced
- ¼ teaspoon red pepper flakes
- 8 black peppercorns
- 6 coriander seeds

Directions:

Divide asparagus, onions, dill, cloves, garlic, pepper flakes, coriander and peppercorns into jars. In a bowl, mix apple cider vinegar with wine vinegar and water and stir well. Divide this into the jars as well, put the lid on and seal. Keep jars in a cold place for 4 weeks before you serve it as a snack. Enjoy!

Nutrition: calories 30, fat 0, fiber 2, carbs 4, protein 2

Delicious Ceviche

Everyone will adore this elegant dash diet appetizer!

Preparation time: 3 hours and 10 minutes
Cooking time: 6 minutes
Servings: 8

Ingredients:

- ¼ pound shrimp, peeled, deveined and chopped
- Zest and juice of 2 limes
- Zest and juice of 2 lemons
- 2 teaspoons cumin, ground
- 2 tablespoons olive oil
- 1 cup tomato, chopped
- ½ cup red onion, chopped
- 2 tablespoons garlic, minced
- 1 Serrano chili pepper, chopped
- 1 cup black beans, canned and drained
- 1 cup cucumber, chopped
- ¼ cup cilantro, chopped

Directions:

In a bowl, mix lime juice and lemon juice with shrimp, toss well, cover and keep in the fridge for 3 hours. Heat up a pan with the oil over medium high heat, add shrimp and citrus juices, cook for 2 minutes on each side and transfer everything to a bowl. Add lime and lemon zest, cumin, tomato, onion, garlic, chili pepper, cucumber, black beans and cilantro, toss well and serve with some tortilla chips on the side. Enjoy!

Nutrition: calories 100, fat 3, fiber 2, carbs 10, protein 5

Simple Marinated Shrimp

This appetizer will surprise you for sure!

Preparation time: 1 hour and 10 minutes
Cooking time: 2 minutes
Servings: 8

Ingredients:

- 2 tablespoons capers
- ½ cup lime juice
- 1 red onion, chopped
- ½ teaspoon hot sauce
- 1 tablespoon mustard
- ½ cup rice vinegar
- 1 cup water
- 1 bay leaf
- 3 cloves
- 1 pound shrimp, peeled and deveined

Directions:

In a baking dish, mix capers with mustard, lime juice and hot sauce and whisk well. Put the water in a pot and heat up over medium heat. Add cloves, bay leaf and vinegar, stir and bring to a boil. Add shrimp, cook for 1 minute, drain and transfer shrimp to the baking dish. Toss to coat well, cover and keep in the fridge fro 1 hour. Divide into bowls and serve. Enjoy!

Nutrition: calories 50, fat 0, fiber 1, carbs 3, protein 12

Delicious Red Pepper Spread

This looks incredible but it tastes divine!

Preparation time: 10 minutes
Cooking time: 0 minutes
Servings: 16

Ingredients:

- 1 cup red bell pepper, roasted and sliced
- 1 tablespoon olive oil
- 2 tablespoons white sesame seeds
- 2 cups canned chickpeas, drained
- 1 tablespoon lemon juice
- 1 teaspoon garlic powder
- 1 teaspoon onion powder
- A pinch of sea salt
- A pinch of cayenne pepper
- 1 and ¼ teaspoons cumin, ground

Directions:

In your food processor, mix red bell pepper with oil, sesame seeds, chickpeas, lemon juice, garlic and onion powder, salt, cayenne pepper and cumin and pulse really well. Divide into serving bowls and serve cold. Enjoy!

Nutrition: calories 50, fat 2, fiber 2, carbs 7, protein 3

Tasty Trout Spread

A smoked trout spread is much more delicious than any other fish spread!

Preparation time: 10 minutes
Cooking time: 0 minutes
Servings: 12

Ingredients:

- ½ cup low fat cottage cheese
- ¼ pound smoked trout fillet, skinless and flaked
- 2 teaspoons lemon juice
- ¼ cup red onion, chopped
- 1 teaspoon hot pepper sauce
- 1 celery stick, chopped
- ½ teaspoon Worcestershire sauce

Directions:

In your food processor, mix trout with cheese, lemon juice, onion, pepper sauce, celery and Worcestershire sauce and blend well. Transfer to a bowl and keep in the fridge until you serve it. Enjoy!

Nutrition: calories 40, fat 1, fiber 0, carbs 1, protein 5

Special White Bean Dip

This is rich and extremely flavored!

Preparation time: 10 minutes
Cooking time: 0 minutes
Servings: 8

Ingredients:

- 15 ounces canned white beans, drained
- 2 tablespoons olive oil
- 8 garlic cloves, roasted in the oven at 350 degrees F for 40 minutes
- 2 tablespoons lemon juice

Directions:

In your food processor, mix beans with oil, garlic and lemon juice and blend well. Divide into bowls and serve this dip with red bell pepper strips on the side. Enjoy!

Nutrition: calories 89, fat 4, fiber 3, carbs 7, protein 2

Spinach and Mint Dip

The mint gives this dash diet dip such a special flavor!

Preparation time: 20 minutes
Cooking time: 0 minutes
Servings: 4

Ingredients:

- 1 bunch spinach leaves, roughly chopped
- 1 scallion, sliced
- 2 tablespoons mint leaves, chopped
- ¾ cup low fat sour cream
- Black pepper to the taste

Directions:

Put spinach in boiling water over medium heat, cook for 20 seconds, rinse and drain well, chop finely and put in a bowl. Add sour cream, scallion, pepper to the taste and of course, the mint, stir well, leave aside for 15 minutes and then serve with pita chips. Enjoy!

Nutrition: calories 140, fat 3, fiber 3, carbs 6, protein 5

Dash Diet Fish and Seafood Recipes

Scallops and Prosciutto

You only need a few special ingredients in order to prepare an elegant and delicious dash diet seafood dish!

Preparation time: 10 minutes
Cooking time: 5 minutes
Servings: 12

Ingredients:

- 2 pounds scallops
- 1 pound prosciutto, sliced
- Some olive oil
- 2 lemons, cut in wedges
- A pinch of salt and some black pepper

Direction:

Cut each prosciutto slice in half, fold lengthwise and wrap each scallop. Sprinkle salt and black pepper on each scallop and prosciutto wrap. Drizzle some olive oil on the scallops as well. Heat up you kitchen grill over medium high heat and grill scallops for 3 minutes on each side. Squeeze 1 lemon wedge on scallops, divide them between plates and serve right away with the rest of the lemon wedges. Enjoy!

Nutrition: calories 140, fat 2, fiber 2, carbs 7, protein 7

Delicious Mussels and Chorizo

You will discover and unique taste and a rich texture!

Preparation time: 10 minutes
Cooking time: 30 minutes
Servings: 4

Ingredients:

- 3 tablespoons olive oil
- 2 pounds mussels, already scrubbed
- 4 ounces dried chorizo, sliced
- Black pepper to the taste
- 3 cups canned tomatoes, crushed with sauce
- 1 big shallot, minced
- 2 garlic cloves, minced
- ¼ teaspoon red pepper flakes, crushed
- 2 cups dry white wine
- 1/3 cup parsley, chopped

Directions:

Heat up a large pan with the olive oil over medium high heat, add shallots, stir and cook for 3 minutes. Add garlic and red pepper flakes, stir and cook for another 3 minutes. Add wine, bring to a boil, reduce heat, crushed tomatoes with sauce and chorizo, stir and boil for 15 minutes Add black pepper and mussels, cover pan, reduce heat to low and simmer for 10 minutes Add parsley at the end, stir and serve right away! Enjoy!

Nutrition: calories 150, fat 2, fiber 3, carbs 10, protein 4

Shrimp Cocktail

This is a popular dish! Try it soon!

Preparation time: 10 minutes
Cooking time: 5 minutes
Servings: 8

Ingredients:

- 2 pounds big shrimp, deveined
- 4 cup water
- 2 bay leaves
- 1 small lemon, halved
- Ice for cooling the shrimp
- Ice for serving
- 1 medium lemon sliced for serving
- ¾ cup ketchup
- 2 and ½ tablespoons horseradish, prepared
- ¼ teaspoon hot pepper sauce
- 2 tablespoons lemon juice

Directions:

Pour the 4 cups water in a large pot, add lemon and bay leaves, Bring to a boil over medium high heat, reduce temperature and boil for 10 minutes. Add shrimp, stir and cook for 2 minutes. Transfer shrimp to a bowl filled with ice and leave aside for 5 minutes. In a bowl, mix ketchup with horseradish and hot pepper sauce and lemon juice and stir well. Place shrimp in a serving bowl filled with ice, with lemon slices and serve with the cocktail sauce you've prepared. Enjoy!

Nutrition: calories 140, fat 1, fiber 3, carbs 10, protein 2

Quinoa and Scallops Salad

You will enjoy some special textures and flavors if you decide to try this salad!

Preparation time: 10 minutes
Cooking time: 35 minutes
Servings: 6

Ingredients:

- 12 ounces dry sea scallops
- 4 tablespoons canola oil
- 2 teaspoons canola oil
- 4 teaspoons low sodium soy sauce
- 1 and ½ cup quinoa, rinsed
- 2 teaspoons garlic, minced
- 3 cups water
- 1 cup snow peas, sliced diagonally
- 1 teaspoon sesame oil
- 1/3 cup rice vinegar
- 1 cup scallions, sliced
- 1/3 cup red bell pepper, chopped
- ¼ cup cilantro, chopped

Directions:

In a bowl, mix scallops with 2 teaspoons soy sauce, stir gently and leave aside for now. Heat up a pan with 1 tablespoon canola oil over medium high heat, add the quinoa, stir and cook for 8 minutes. Add garlic, stir and cook for 1 more minute. Add the water, bring to a boil over medium heat, stir, cover and cook for 15 minutes. Remove from heat and leave aside covered for 5 minutes. Add snow peas, cover again and leave for 5 more minutes. Meanwhile, in a bowl, mix 3 tablespoons canola oil with 2 teaspoons soy sauce, vinegar and sesame oil and stir well. Add quinoa and snow peas to this mixture and stir again. Add scallions, bell pepper and stir again. Pat dry the scallops and discard marinade. Heat up another pan with 2 teaspoons canola oil over high heat, add scallops and cook for 1 minute on each side. Add them to the quinoa salad, stir gently and serve with chopped cilantro.

Nutrition: calories 150, fat 1, fiber 2, carbs 8, protein 4

Squid and Shrimp Salad

This is easy to make and it's so healthy!

Preparation time: 10 minutes
Cooking time: 15 minutes
Servings: 4

Ingredients:

- 8 ounces squid, cut into medium pieces
- 8 ounces shrimp, peeled and deveined
- 1 red onion, sliced
- 1 cucumber, chopped
- 2 tomatoes, cut into medium wedges
- 2 tablespoons cilantro, chopped
- 1 hot jalapeno pepper, cut in rounds
- 3 tablespoons rice vinegar
- 3 tablespoons dark sesame oil
- Black pepper to the taste

Method:

In a bowl, mix onion with cucumber, tomatoes, pepper, cilantro, shrimp and squid and stir well. Cut a big parchment paper in half, fold it in half heart shape and open. Place the seafood mixture in this parchment piece, fold over, seal edges, place on a baking sheet and introduce in the oven at 400 degrees F for 15 minutes. Meanwhile, in a small bowl mix sesame oil with rice vinegar and black pepper and stir very well. Take the salad out of the oven, leave to cool down for a few minutes and transfer to a serving plate. Drizzle the dressing over the salad and serve right away. Enjoy!

Nutrition: calories 150, fat 1, fiber 4, carbs 15, protein 3

Popular Seafood Salad

You will love this very simple seafood salad!

Preparation time: 2 hours and 10 minutes
Cooking time: 1 hour and 30 minutes
Servings: 4
Ingredients:

- 1 big octopus, cleaned
- 1 pound mussels
- 2 pounds clams
- 1 big squid cut in rings
- 3 garlic cloves, chopped
- 1 celery rib, cut crosswise into thirds
- ½ cup celery rib, sliced
- 1 carrot, cut crosswise into 3 pieces
- 1 small white onion, chopped
- 1 bay leaf
- ¾ cup white wine
- 2 cups radicchio, sliced
- 1 red onion, sliced
- 1 cup parsley, chopped
- 1 cup olive oil
- 1 cup red wine vinegar
- Black pepper to the taste

Directions:

Place the octopus in a large pot with celery rib cut in thirds, garlic, carrot, bay leaf, white onion and white wine. Add water to cover the octopus, cover with a lid, bring to a boil over high heat, reduce temperature to low and simmer for 1 and ½ hours. Drain octopus, reserve boiling liquid and leave aside to cool down. Put ¼ cup octopus cooking liquid in another pot, add mussels, heat up over medium high heat, cook until they open, transfer to a bowl and leave aside. Add clams to the pan, cover, cook over medium high heat until they open, transfer to the bowl with mussels and leave aside. Add squid to the pan, cover and cook over medium high heat for 3 minutes, transfer to the bowl with mussels and clams. Meanwhile, slice octopus into small pieces and mix with the rest of the seafood. Add sliced celery, radicchio, red onion, vinegar, olive oil, parsley, salt and pepper, stir gently and leave aside in the fridge for 2 hours before serving. Enjoy!

Nutrition: calories 200, fat 4, fiber 4, carbs 14, protein 2

Shrimp and Delicious Ginger Dressing

A delicious salad topped with the best ginger dressing is just what you need today

Preparation time: 10 minutes
Cooking time: 5 minutes
Servings: 2

Ingredients:

- 8 medium shrimp, peeled and deveined
- 12 ounces package mixed salad leaves
- 10 cherry tomatoes, halved
- 2 green onions, sliced
- 2 medium mushrooms, sliced
- 1/3 cup rice vinegar
- ¼ cup sesame seeds, toasted
- 1 tablespoon low sodium soy sauce
- 2 teaspoons ginger, grated
- 2 teaspoons garlic, minced
- 2/3 cup canola oil
- 1/3 cup sesame oil

Directions:

In a bowl, mix rice vinegar with sesame seeds, soy sauce, garlic, ginger and stir well. Pour this into your kitchen blender, add canola oil and sesame oil, pulse very well and leave aside. Brush shrimp with 3 tablespoons of the ginger dressing you've prepared. Heat up your kitchen grill over high heat, add shrimp and cook for 3 minutes flipping once. In a salad bowl, mix salad leaves with grilled shrimp, mushrooms, green onions and tomatoes. Drizzle ginger dressing on top and serve right away! Enjoy!

Nutrition: calories 140, fat 1, fiber 3, carbs 7, protein 4

Delicious Shrimp Soup

Enjoy this amazing soup as soon as possible!

Preparation time: 10 minutes
Cooking time: 25 minutes
Servings: 6

Ingredients:

- 8 ounces shrimp, peeled and deveined
- 1 stalk lemongrass, smashed
- 2 small ginger pieces, grated
- 6 cup chicken stock
- 2 jalapenos, chopped
- 4 lime leaves
- 1 and ½ cups pineapple, chopped
- 1 cup shiitake mushroom caps, chopped
- 1 tomato, chopped
- ½ bell pepper, cubed
- 2 tablespoons fish sauce
- 1 teaspoon sugar
- ¼ cup lime juice
- 1/3 cup cilantro, chopped
- 2 scallions, sliced

Directions:

In a pot mix ginger with lemongrass, stock, jalapenos and lime leaves, stir, bring to a boil over medium heat, cover and cook for 15 minutes. Strain liquid in a bowl and discard solids. Return soup to the pot again, add pineapple, tomato, mushrooms, bell pepper, sugar and fish sauce, stir, bring to a boil over medium heat, cook for 5 minutes, add shrimp and cook for 3 more minutes. Remove from heat, add lime juice, cilantro and scallions, stir, ladle into soup bowls and serve. Enjoy!

Nutrition: calories 140, fat 2, fiber 3, carbs 15, protein 3

Mussels And Chickpea Soup

This exotic soup will be perfect for a very hot summer day!

Preparation time: 10 minutes
Cooking time: 10 minutes
Servings: 6

Ingredients:

- 3 garlic cloves, minced
- 2 tablespoons olive oil
- A pinch of chili flakes
- 1 and ½ tablespoons fresh mussels, scrubbed
- 1 cup white wine
- 1 cup chickpeas, rinsed
- 1 small fennel bulb, sliced
- Black pepper to the taste
- Juice of 1 lemon
- 3 tablespoons parsley, chopped

Directions:

Heat up a big saucepan with the olive oil over medium high heat, add garlic and chili flakes, stir and cook for a couple of minutes. Add white wine and mussels, stir, cover and cook for 3-4 minutes until mussels open. Transfer mussels to a baking dish, add some of the cooking liquid over them and keep in the fridge until they are cold enough. Take mussels out of the fridge and discard shells. Heat up another pan over medium high heat, add mussels, reserved cooking liquid, chickpeas and fennel, stir well and heat them up Add black pepper to the taste, lemon juice and parsley, stir again, divide between plates and serve. Enjoy!

Nutrition: calories 150, fat 3, fiber 6, carbs 20, protein 4

Gourmet Salmon Delight

This is a special, elegant and super delicious dash diet salmon dish!

Preparation time: 15 minutes
Cooking time: 20 minutes
Servings: 6

Ingredients:

- 2 untreated cedar planks
- 1/3 cup vegetable oil
- 1 and ½ tablespoons rice vinegar
- 1/3 cup low sodium soy sauce
- 1 teaspoon sesame oil
- ¼ cup green onions, chopped
- 1 teaspoon garlic, minced
- 1 tablespoon ginger, grated
- 2 salmon fillets, skinless and boneless

Directions:

Place cedar planks in a dish, cover with warm water and soak for about 1 hour. Meanwhile, in an another dish mix vegetable oil with vinegar, soy sauce, sesame oil, ginger, green onions and garlic and whisk well Add salmon to this mix, cover and leave aside for 15 minutes. Heat up your grill over medium heat, place planks on it and add salmon fillets when planks begin to smoke. Cover grill and cook for 20 minutes. Divide between plates and serve right away! Enjoy!

Nutrition: calories 240, fat 3, fiber 3, carbs 20, protein 5

Scallops and Jalapeno Vinaigrette

This is one of the most incredible dash diet dishes you'll ever have!

Preparation time: 5 minutes
Cooking time: 6 minutes
Servings: 4

Ingredients:

- 1 jalapeno pepper, seedless and minced
- ¼ cup extra virgin olive oil
- ¼ cup rice vinegar
- ¼ teaspoon mustard
- Black pepper to the taste
- A pinch cayenne pepper
- 1 tablespoon vegetable oil
- 12 big sea scallops
- 2 oranges, sliced

Directions:

In your blender, mix jalapeno with olive oil, mustard, black and vinegar and pulse really well. Season scallops with cayenne pepper. Heat up a pan with the vegetable oil over high temperature, add scallops and cook them for 3 minutes on each side. Divide scallops on plates, place orange slices on top and drizzle the jalapeno vinaigrette. Enjoy!

Nutrition: calories 150, fat 1, fiber 2, carbs 8, protein 4

Broiled Lobster Tails

This is a great dish perfect for every special occasion!

Preparation time: 10 minutes
Cooking time: 10 minutes
Servings: 2

Ingredients:

- 2 big whole lobster tails
- ½ teaspoon paprika
- ½ cup coconut butter
- White pepper to the taste
- 1 lemon cut in wedges

Directions

Place lobster tails on a baking sheet, cut top side of lobster shells and pull them apart Season with white pepper and paprika. Add butter and toss gently Introduce lobster tails in preheated broiler and broil for 10 minutes. Divide on plates, garnish with lemon wedges and serve right away! Enjoy!

Nutrition: calories 140, fat 2, fiber 2, carbs 6, protein 6

Tuna and Orange Salsa

This is truly a summer dish for you to try as soon as possible!

Preparation time: 10 minutes
Cooking time: 5 minutes
Servings: 4

Ingredients:

- 2 oranges, sliced
- ½ cup red onion, chopped
- 1 red bell pepper, chopped
- ¼ cup mint, chopped
- 1 tablespoon red wine vinegar
- 1 tablespoon vegetable oil
- Black pepper to the taste
- 4 tuna steaks
- 1 teaspoon coriander, dried

Directions:

In a bowl, mix oranges with onion, bell pepper, mint, vinegar, salt and pepper, stir and leave aside for now. Heat up your kitchen grill over medium high heat, rub tuna steaks with oil, pepper and coriander and grill for about 5 minutes. Divide on plates, top with the orange salsa you've prepared and serve. Enjoy!

Nutrition: calories 140, fat 2, fiber 3, carbs 9, protein 4

Delicious Seafood Stew

You can prepare this simple recipe for lunch and even for a fast dinner!

Preparation time: 10 minutes
Cooking time: 12 minutes
Servings: 4

Ingredients:

- 12 jumbo shrimp, peeled (shells reserved) and deveined
- 4 parsley springs
- ¼ cup parsley, chopped
- 1 garlic clove, minced
- 1 tablespoon garlic, minced
- 1 tablespoon extra virgin olive oil
- ¼ cup shallot, chopped
- 1 cup dry white wine
- 2 dozen clams, scrubbed
- 1 pound mussels, scrubbed
- Black pepper to the taste
- 1 tomato, chopped
- 8 scallops halved horizontally
- 2 cups water

Directions:

Heat up a pan over high heat, add shrimp shells and 1 garlic clove, stir and cook for 2 minutes. Add parsley springs and water, stir, bring to a boil, cook for 3 minutes, strain into a bowl and leave aside for now. Meanwhile, heat up another pan with the olive oil over medium high heat, add 1 tablespoon garlic and shallots, stir and cook for 1 minute. Add wine and shrimp stock, add clams and mussels, bring to a simmer and cook for 4 minutes until clams open. Divide clams and mussels into bowls, sprinkle chopped parsley and leave aside. Season broth with black pepper, add scallops, shrimp and tomato, cover and cook for 2 more minutes over medium heat. Add this mix to the bowls with the clams and mussels sprinkle chopped parsley and serve. Enjoy!

Nutrition: calories 150, fat 2, fiber 3, carbs 7, protein 3

Healthy Steamed Fish

If you are looking for a very healthy dash diet fish dish, then this is definitely the right one!

Preparation time: 10 minutes
Cooking time: 10 minutes
Servings: 4

Ingredients:
- 4 white fish fillets
- 1 tablespoon olive oil
- 1 teaspoon thyme, dried
- 1 pound cherry tomatoes, halved
- 1 cup black olives, pitted and chopped
- A pinch of sea salt and black pepper
- 1 garlic clove, minced
- 1 cup water

Directions:
Put the water in your instant pot, place the steamer basket on top and arrange fish inside. Season with salt, pepper, thyme and garlic. Add oil, olives and tomatoes, rub gently, cover your instant pot and cook on Low for 10 minutes. Release the pressure fast, divide fish and all veggies between plates and serve hot. Enjoy!

Nutrition: calories 140, fat 2, fiber 2, carbs 8, protein 2

Shrimp Umani

Enjoy a different and exotic dash diet shrimp dish!

Preparation time: 10 minutes
Cooking time: 3 minutes
Servings: 2

Ingredients:
- 8 big shrimp
- 1 tablespoon ginger, grated
- 3 tablespoons low sodium soy sauce
- 1/3 cup sake
- 1 cup dashi
- 3 tablespoons mirin
- 1 tablespoon sugar

Directions:
Heat up a pan with the dashi over medium heat, add sugar, ginger, soy sauce, mirin and sake, stir and bring to a boil. Add shrimp, cook for 3 minutes, take off heat, leave aside to cool down completely, divide between 2 plates and serve. Enjoy!

Nutrition: calories 100, fat 1, fiber 3, carbs 6, protein 3

Simple Herring Roe

This herring roe is much more delicious than you can imagine!

Preparation time: 10 minutes
Cooking time: 5 minutes
Servings: 4

Ingredients:

- 10 pieces herring roe, soaked in water for half a day and drained
- 3 cups water
- Kombu, thinly sliced
- 3 tablespoons mirin
- 3 tablespoons sake
- 6 tablespoons low sodium soy sauce
- 1 teaspoon sugar
- 1 handful bonito flakes

Directions:

In a pot, mix water with kombu, mirin, sake, soy sauce and sugar, stir and bring to a boil over medium heat. Add herring roe, cook for 2 minutes, take off heat and add bonito flakes. Leave everything to cool down in the pot, divide herring roe into bowls and serve. Enjoy!

Nutrition: calories 140, fat 2, fiber 3, carbs 6, protein 3

Mexican Shrimp Salad

Are you in the mood for a healthy and light seafood salad? Try this dash diet one!

Preparation time: 10 minutes
Cooking time: 20 minutes
Servings: 6

Ingredients:

- 1 pound shrimp, deveined and peeled
- 2 cups cherry tomatoes, halved
- 2 romaine lettuce hearts, shredded
- 1 cucumber, chopped
- 1 avocado, pitted, peeled and chopped
- ½ cup cilantro leaves, chopped
- Black pepper to the taste
- 4 cups tortilla chips
- 2 tablespoons low fat sour cream
- 2 tablespoons lime juice
- ½ teaspoon lime zest, grated

Directions:

Put water in a pot, bring to a boil over medium high heat, add shrimp, cook for 3 minutes, transfer them to a bowl filled with ice water, drain, pat dry them and put in a salad bowl. Add lettuce, cucumber, tomatoes, avocado, cilantro and tortilla chips. In a bowl, mix sour cream with lime juice, lime zest, and black pepper to the taste and whisk well. Pour this over salad, toss to coat and serve right away. Enjoy!

Nutrition: calories 150, fat 2, fiber 4, carbs 7, protein 3

Special Tuna Kabobs

They look amazing and they taste divine!

Preparation time: 30 minutes
Cooking time: 10 minutes
Servings: 16

Ingredients:

- ¼ cup low sodium soy sauce
- 1 pound tuna steaks, cubed in 16 pieces
- 2 tablespoons rice vinegar
- Black pepper to the taste
- 1 tablespoon sesame seeds
- 2 tablespoons canola oil
- 16 pieces pickled ginger
- 1 bunch watercress

Directions:

In a bowl, mix soy sauce with vinegar and tuna, toss to coat, cover bowl and keep in the fridge for 30 minutes. Discard marinade, pat dry tuna and sprinkle it with black pepper and sesame seeds. Heat up a pan with the oil over medium heat, add tuna pieces, cook them until they are pink in the center and browned on the outside, take them off heat and transfer them to a plate. Thread one ginger slice on 16 skewers. Thread one tuna cube on each of the 16 skewers. Arrange watercress on a platter, arrange tuna kabobs on top and serve. Enjoy!

Nutrition: calories 150, fat 1, fiber 4, carbs 19, protein 4

Roasted Salmon

This will impress your family for sure!

Preparation time: 10 minutes
Cooking time: 35 minutes
Servings: 6

Ingredients:

- 2 pounds salmon fillets, boneless
- 1 garlic clove, minced
- ¼ cup maple syrup
- ¼ cup balsamic vinegar
- A pinch of black pepper
- Chopped mint for serving
- Cooking spray

Directions:

Heat up a pan over medium low heat, add maple syrup, vinegar and garlic, stir and heat up for 1 minutes. Transfer this to a bowl and leave aside to cool down a bit. Spray a baking sheet with cooking spray, arrange salmon fillets on the sheet, season them with a pinch of black pepper and brush with half of the maple glaze. Introduce in the oven at 450 degrees F and bake for 10 minutes. Brush salmon with the rest of the glaze and bake for 20 minutes more. Divide on plates, sprinkle mint on top and serve. Enjoy!

Nutrition: calories 180, fat 2, fiber 4, carbs 10, protein 4

Amazing Baked Chicken

This is so flavored and tasty!

Preparation time: 40 minutes
Cooking time: 1 hour and 10 minutes
Servings: 6

Ingredients:
- 1 and ½ cups celery, chopped
- 1 pound chicken breast halves, skinless, boneless and cut into medium pieces
- 1 and ½ cups pearl onions
- 2 cups chicken stock
- 1 teaspoon tarragon, chopped
- ¾ cup white rice
- 1 and ½ cups white wine
- ¾ cup wild rice

Directions:
Put half of the stock in a pot, add chicken, tarragon, onions and celery, stir, bring to a simmer over medium heat, cook for 10 minutes, take off heat and leave aside to cool down. In a baking dish, mix the rest of the stock with white and wild rice, stir and leave aside for 30 minutes. Add chicken and the veggies, cover, introduce in the oven at 300 degrees F and bake for 1 hour. Divide between plates and serve right away. Enjoy!

Nutrition: Calories 300, fat 1, fiber 2, carbs 20, protein 20

Simple Roasted Chicken

This roasted chicken is just perfect and it follows the dash diet principles!

Preparation time: 10 minutes
Cooking time: 1 hour and 30 minutes
Servings: 8

Ingredients:
- 1 chicken
- 1 garlic clove, minced
- 1 tablespoon rosemary, chopped
- 1 tablespoon olive oil
- Black pepper to the taste
- ½ cup balsamic vinegar
- 1 teaspoon brown sugar
- 8 rosemary springs

Directions:
In a bowl, mix garlic with rosemary and stir. Rub chicken with black pepper, the oil and rosemary mix, place it in a roasting pan, introduce in the oven at 350 degrees F and roast for 1 hour and 20 minutes basting with pan juices from time to time. Meanwhile, heat up a pan with the vinegar over medium heat, add sugar, stir and cook until it dissolves. Carve chicken and divide between plates. Serve with the vinegar mix and with rosemary springs on top. Enjoy!

Nutrition: calories 345, fat 5, fiber 1, carbs 5, protein 24

Chicken Breast Delight

Make sure you have enough for all your guests!

Preparation time: 1 hour and 10 minutes
Cooking time: 10 minutes
Servings: 6

Ingredients:

- ½ teaspoon canola oil
- 4 garlic cloves, minced
- 1 cup onion, chopped
- 1 cup already cooked brown rice
- 1 pound chicken breast, ground
- 1 teaspoon sweet paprika
- Black pepper to the taste
- 2 teaspoons fennel seeds
- 1 teaspoon cumin seeds
- ½ teaspoon white pepper
- A pinch of cayenne pepper
- 1 teaspoon rosemary, chopped
- 1 teaspoon mustard seeds
- ¼ teaspoon nutmeg, ground
- 1 teaspoon celery seed

Directions:

Heat up a pan with the oil over medium high heat, add onion and garlic, stir and sauté for 3 minutes. In a bowl, mix chicken with cooked rice, onion and garlic, black, white and cayenne pepper, paprika, fennel, cumin, rosemary, celery seeds, mustard seeds and rosemary, stir well and keep in the fridge for 1 hour. Shape rolls out of this mix, place on a lined baking sheet and bake in the oven at 350 degrees F for 20 minutes. Serve hot. Enjoy!

Nutrition: calories 150, fat 1, fiber 2, carbs 12, protein 17

Light Caesar Salad

It's a healthy option for lunch or even for dinner!

Preparation time: 10 minutes
Cooking time: 12 minutes
Servings: 4

Ingredients:

- 1 pound chicken breast, boneless, skinless and cut in halves
- Cooking spray
- Back pepper to the taste
- ½ cup soft tofu, cubed
- 2 tablespoons lemon juice
- 1 and ½ teaspoons mustard
- 1 tablespoon olive oil
- 1 and ½ teaspoons red wine vinegar
- ¾ teaspoon garlic, minced
- 1 tablespoon water
- 1 teaspoon Worcestershire sauce
- 8 cups lettuce leaves, cut in strips
- 4 tablespoons low fat parmesan, grated
- 1 and ¼ cups croutons

Directions:

Spray chicken breasts with some cooking spray and season black pepper to the taste. Heat up you kitchen grill over medium high heat, add chicken breasts, cook for 6 minutes on each side, transfer to a cutting board, leave to cool down for 5 minutes, cut into small pieces, transfer to a bowl and leave aside. In your blender, mix tofu with lemon juice, olive oil, mustard, vinegar, Worcestershire sauce and garlic and blend very well. Add the water and pulse a few more times. Add half of the parmesan and blend some more. In a salad bowl, mix lettuce with chicken and croutons. Pour salad dressing, toss to coat, sprinkle with the rest of the parmesan and serve. Enjoy!

Nutrition: calories 150, fat 2, fiber 3, carbs 9, protein 5

Simple Chicken Salad

You will adore a Mediterranean style salad!

Preparation time: 10 minutes
Cooking time: 0 minutes
Servings: 4

Ingredients:

- 15 ounces canned chickpeas, drained
- 9 ounces chicken breast, already cooked and chopped
- 1 cucumber, chopped
- 4 green onions, chopped
- Black pepper to the taste
- ½ cup fat free yogurt
- ¼ cup mint, chopped
- 2 cups baby spinach
- 2 garlic cloves, minced
- 1/3 cup low fat feta cheese, crumbled
- 4 lemon wedges

Directions:

In a salad bowl, mix chicken meat with chickpeas, cucumber, onions, mint, garlic, salt and pepper. Add yogurt and toss to coat. Add spinach and feta cheese and toss again gently. Serve with lemon wedges on the side. Enjoy!

Nutrition: calories 140, fat 1, fiber 4, carbs 8, protein 2

Chicken and Peanut Sauce

You will enjoy a rich and hearty salad for sure!

Preparation time: 10 minutes
Cooking time: 0 minutes
Servings: 6

Ingredients:

- 4 cups chicken, cooked, boneless, skinless and shredded
- ¼ cup olive oil
- 1/3 cup rice wine vinegar
- 2 teaspoons sesame oil
- ¼ cup already made vegan peanut sauce
- ½ napa cabbage head, shredded
- 1 cup carrot, grated
- 6 scallions, sliced
- Black pepper to the taste
- 2 teaspoons sesame seeds

Directions:

In a bowl, mix olive oil with peanut sauce, vinegar and sesame oil and whisk very well. In a salad bowl, mix chicken with 4 scallions, cabbage and carrot. Add peanut dressing and pepper and toss to coat. Divide on serving plates, sprinkle sesame seeds and the other scallions on top and serve right away. Enjoy!

Nutrition: calories 150, fat 2, fiber 2, carbs 8, protein 6

Special Chicken Salad

We can assure you that this dash diet salad is really tasty!

Preparation time: 10 minutes
Cooking time: 20 minutes
Servings: 2

Ingredients:

- 2 tablespoons olive oil
- 2 ounces quinoa
- 2 ounces cherry tomatoes, cut in quarters
- 3 ounces sweet corn, frozen
- A handful coriander, chopped
- Lime juice from 1 lime
- Lime zest from 1 lime, grated
- Black pepper to the taste
- 2 spring onions, sliced
- ½ red chili pepper, chopped
- 1 avocado, pitted, peeled and chopped
- 7 ounces chicken meat, roasted, skinless, boneless and chopped

Directions:

Put some water in a pan, place on stove and bring to a boil over medium high heat. Add quinoa, stir and cook for 12 minutes. Meanwhile, put corn in a pan, heat up over medium high heat, cook for 5 minutes stirring from time to time, take off heat and leave aside for now. Transfer cooked quinoa to a colander, rinse well, drain and transfer to a bowl. Add tomatoes, corn, coriander, onions, chili, lime zest, olive oil and black pepper to the taste. In another bowl, mix avocado with lime juice and stir well. Mix this with tomatoes and quinoa salad, add chicken, toss to coat and serve. Enjoy!

Nutrition: calories 130, fat 2, fiber 3, carbs 8, protein 7

Delightful Chicken and Eggplant Sandwich

It's going to give you so much energy and it will make you feel full all day long!

Preparation time: 10 minutes
Cooking time: 10 minutes
Servings: 4

Ingredients:

- 4 chicken breasts
- Cooking spray
- A pinch of Italian seasoning
- 1 eggplant, thinly sliced
- Black pepper to the taste
- A drizzle of olive oil
- ½ cup low sodium marinara sauce
- 16 basil leaves, torn
- 8 ounces low fat mozzarella cheese, shredded
- 8 whole wheat bread slices

Directions:

Spray chicken pieces with cooking oil, season with black pepper to the taste and sprinkle Italian seasoning. Heat up a grill over medium high heat, add chicken, cook for 5 minutes on each side, take off heat and leave aside for now. Season eggplant slices with salt to the taste, leave them aside for 10 minutes, drain with paper towels, drizzle extra virgin olive oil over them, season with black pepper to the taste, arrange them on heated grill and cook them until they become soft. Arrange 2 bread slices on a working surface, place 1 ounce mozzarella cheese on each bread slice, add 2 eggplant slices on one slice, 1 grilled chicken piece, 2 tablespoon marinara sauce, 4 basil leaves and top with the other bread slice. Repeat this with the rest of the bread slices, making 4 sandwiches. Heat up your Panini press over high heat, place sandwiches, cook them for 4 minutes, leave them to cool down for 3 minutes, arrange on plates and serve them right away. Enjoy!

Nutrition: calories 140, fat 2, fiber 6, carbs 14, protein 6

Healthy Chicken Wrap

These dash diet wraps look incredible and they taste even better!

Preparation time: 10 minutes
Cooking time: 13 minutes
Servings: 4

Ingredients:

- 4 chicken breast halves, skinless and boneless
- Black pepper to the taste
- 4 teaspoons olive oil
- ½ cucumber, sliced lengthwise
- 3 teaspoons cilantro, chopped
- 4 whole wheat tortillas
- 4 tablespoons vegan peanut sauce

Directions:

Mix chicken with the oil and season with black pepper. Heat up your grill over medium high heat, add chicken, cook for 6 minutes on each side, transfer to a cutting board, leave to cool down for 5 minutes, slice and leave aside. In a bowl, mix cilantro with cucumber and stir. Heat up a pan over medium heat, add each tortilla, heat up for 20 seconds and transfer them to a working surface. Spread 1 tablespoon peanut sauce on each tortilla, divide chicken and cucumber mix on each, fold, arrange on plates and serve. Enjoy!

Nutrition: calories 150, fat 1, fiber 2, carbs 6, protein 7

Simple Chicken Wraps

It's a very simple recipe but a very rich one at the same time and the best thing is that it's 100% dash diet!

Preparation time: 10 minutes
Cooking time: 0 minutes
Servings: 4

Ingredients:

- 4 whole wheat tortillas
- 1/3 cup fat free yogurt
- 6 ounces chicken breasts, cooked and cut into thin strips
- 2 tomatoes, chopped
- ¾ cup cucumber, sliced very thinly
- Black pepper to the taste

Directions:

Heat up a pan over medium heat, add one tortilla at the time, heat up and arrange them on a working surface. Spread yogurt on each. Add chicken, cucumber and tomatoes. Roll tortillas, arrange them on plates and serve right away. Enjoy!

Nutrition: calories 100, fat 1, fiber 2, carbs 6, protein 4

Healthy and Delicious Chicken Soup

It's so flavored and tasty! Just make sure you get all the right ingredients and follow all the directions!

Preparation time: 10 minutes
Cooking time: 2 hours
Servings: 6

Ingredients:

- 1 whole chicken, cut into medium pieces
- 6 celery stalks, chopped
- 6 carrots, sliced
- 1 onion, halved
- A bunch parsley springs
- A bunch dill springs
- 2 tablespoons dill, chopped
- 3 cloves
- 2 tablespoons black peppercorns
- A pinch of black pepper
- 2 bay leaves
- ¼ teaspoon saffron threads

Directions:

Put chicken pieces in a pot, add water to cover, place on stove, bring to a boil over medium high heat, cook for 15 minutes and skim foam well. Add celery, onion, carrots, parsley springs, dill springs, whole cloves, bay leaves, peppercorns and some black pepper, stir, cover pot, reduce heat to medium- low and simmer for 1 hour and 30 minutes. Take soup off heat, take chicken pieces out and leave them aside to cool down. Strain soup into another pot, reserve carrots and celery but discard herbs and spices. Discard bones from chicken pieces, cut meat into strips and return to pot. Heat up soup with reserved veggies, add chicken pieces, crushed saffron and chopped dill and stir. Pour into soup bowls and serve right away. Enjoy!

Nutrition: calories 140, fat 2, fiber 2, carbs 7, protein 6

Spring Chicken Soup

It's such an easy dash diet recipe that even an amateur can make it at home in no time!

Preparation time: 10 minutes
Cooking time: 35 minutes
Servings: 6

Ingredients:

- 2 chicken breasts, cooked, skinless, boneless and shredded
- 2 bacon slices, chopped
- A pinch of sea salt
- Black pepper to the taste
- 1 and ½ cups mushrooms, chopped
- 1 yellow onion, chopped
- 2 carrots, chopped
- 3 garlic cloves, minced
- 4 cups spinach, torn
- 12 asparagus spears, chopped
- 6 cups low sodium chicken stock
- 15 ounces canned cannellini beans, drained
- 1 and ¼ cups small pasta
- Lime zest from ½ lime, grated
- 1/3 cup low fat parmesan, grated
- ½ handful cilantro, chopped for serving
- 1 avocado, pitted, peeled and chopped very finely for serving
- 3 green onions, finely chopped for serving

Directions:

Heat up a soup pot over medium high heat, add bacon, stir, cook for 2-3 minutes, take off heat, transfer to paper towels, drain fat and return to pot. Add mushrooms and onions to pot, stir and cook for 5 minutes. Add carrots, garlic and asparagus, stir and cook for 5 minutes more. Add spinach, salt and pepper, stir again and cook another 3 minutes. Add stock, chicken meat, beans and pasta, stir, bring to a boil, reduce heat to medium low and simmer for 15 minutes. Add cheese and lime zest, stir and pour into soup bowls. Serve with cilantro, avocado and green onions on top. Enjoy!

Nutrition: calories 150, fat 1, fiber 2, carbs 10, protein 3

Autumn Chicken Cream

This dash diet soup is perfect for a cold autumn day!

Preparation time: 10 minutes
Cooking time: 20 minutes
Servings: 4

Ingredients:

- 2 chicken breasts, cut into strips
- 1 yellow onion, chopped
- 2 tablespoons coconut oil
- 1 garlic clove, chopped
- 12 ounces pumpkin, peeled, seedless and cut in small cubes
- 12 ounces sweet potatoes, chopped
- 2 carrots, chopped
- ½ teaspoon ginger, grated
- ½ teaspoon cumin, ground
- 1 teaspoon turmeric, ground
- Black pepper to the taste
- A pinch of sea salt
- 14 ounces coconut milk
- 17 ounces low sodium chicken stock.

Directions:

Heat up a pot with the oil over medium high heat, add garlic and onion, stir and cook for 2 minutes. Add carrots, pumpkin and potato, stir and cook for 5 minutes. Add ginger, cumin, turmeric, chicken stock, coconut milk and chicken, stir, bring to a boil, reduce heat to medium and simmer for 10 minutes. Add a pinch of salt and pepper to the taste, transfer soup to your blender and pulse twice. Ladle into soup bowls and serve right away. Enjoy!

Nutrition: calories 140, fat 1, fiber 4, carbs 15, protein 2

Chicken and Noodles Soup

It's the best combination ever! Try this soup today!

Preparation time: 10 minutes
Cooking time: 35 minutes
Servings: 8

Ingredients:

- 3 carrots, sliced
- 3 celery stalks, sliced thinly
- 1 tablespoon olive oil
- 1 tablespoon cornstarch
- 1 onion, chopped
- 6 cups low sodium chicken stock
- 1/3 cup water
- 1 pound egg noodles
- 2 teaspoons thyme, chopped
- 2 teaspoons parsley, chopped
- 2 cups chicken meat, already cooked
- Black pepper to the taste
- A pinch of salt
- 4 green onions, chopped

Directions:

Heat up a pot with the oil over medium high heat, add onion, carrots and celery, stir and cook for 6 minutes. Add stock, stir, bring to a boil, reduce heat to medium low and simmer for 20 minutes. In a small bowl, mix cornstarch with the water and stir well. Pour this over soup, add noodles, stir and cook for a few more minutes. Add a pinch of salt and black pepper to the taste, thyme, parsley and chicken meat, stir again well and cook for 3-4 minutes. Ladle soup into bowls, sprinkle sliced green onions on top and serve. Enjoy!

Nutrition: calories 130, fat 1, fiber 3, carbs 6, protein 6

Baked Chicken Wings

Are you looking for something tasty to cook tonight? Try this idea!

Preparation time: 10 minutes
Cooking time: 1 hour and 15 minutes
Servings: 4

Ingredients:

- 2 pounds chicken wings
- 1 tablespoon Italian seasoning
- Black pepper to the taste
- A pinch of salt
- 2 tablespoons olive oil
- 2 tablespoons honey
- 1 and ¼ cups balsamic vinegar
- 3 garlic cloves, minced

Directions:

In a bowl, mix chicken wings with Italian seasoning, salt, pepper and the olive oil and toss to coat. Transfer to a baking dish, introduce in preheated oven at 425 degrees F and bake for 1 hour. Heat up a pan over medium heat, add garlic, vinegar and honey, stir well, bring to a boil and simmer for 10 minutes. Take chicken wings out of the oven, transfer to a bowl, add vinegar glaze, toss to coat and return them to baking dish. Introduce in the oven again, bake for 5 more minutes and then arrange them on a platter. Serve hot. Enjoy!

Nutrition: calories 130, fat 2, fiber 3, carbs 8, protein 3

Chicken with Tasty Salsa

It's perfect for when you don't have time to make something more complex!

Preparation time: 50 minutes
Servings: 4

Ingredients:

- 1 pound chicken breast, boneless and skinless
- 16 ounces canned salsa Verde
- Black pepper to the taste
- A pinch of sea salt
- 1 tablespoon olive oil
- 1 and ½ cups fat free Monterey jack cheese, shredded
- ¼ cup cilantro, chopped
- Wild rice, cooked for serving
- Juice from 1 lime

Directions:

Mix chicken with salt, pepper, and oil and toss to coat. Spread salsa in a baking dish, add chicken on top, introduce in the oven at 400 degrees F and bake for 40 minutes. Take chicken out of the oven, add cheese, introduce everything in preheated broiler and broil for 3 minutes. Add lime juice, divide between plates, sprinkle cilantro and serve with white rice. Enjoy!

Nutrition: calories 150, fat 1, fiber 4, carbs 20, protein 4

Amazing Chicken Casserole

It's simply heavenly! You must really try this recipe tonight!

Preparation time: 10 minutes
Cooking time: 5 minutes
Servings: 8

Ingredients:

- 2 tablespoons olive oil
- 2 pounds chicken breasts, skinless and boneless
- 2 carrots, chopped
- Black pepper to the taste
- 1 yellow onion, chopped
- 1 teaspoon Cajun seasoning
- ¼ cup flour
- ½ cup orange juice
- 1 can low sodium chicken stock
- 1 cup peas
- ½ cup parsley, chopped
- 2 tablespoons dill, chopped
- ½ cup fat free buttermilk
- 2 and ½ cups cornflakes

Directions:

Put water in a pot, add chicken, bring to a boil over medium heat, simmer for 10 minutes, drain and leave aside for now. Heat up a pan with the oil over medium high heat, add onion, carrots and pepper, stir and cook for 10 minutes. Add Cajun seasoning and flour, stir and cook for 1 minute. Add stock and orange juice stirring all the time and bring to a boil. Add chicken, dill, peas and half of the parsley, stir and take off heat. Add buttermilk, stir, transfer everything to a baking dish, introduce in the oven at 375 degrees F and bake for 15 minutes. Meanwhile, in a bowl, mix cornflakes with the rest of the parsley and stir. Take chicken out of the oven, sprinkle cornflakes all over, introduce in the oven again and bake for 6 more minutes. Take dish out of the oven, leave aside for 10 minutes, divide between plates and serve. Enjoy!

Nutrition: calories 130, fat 3, fiber 3, carbs 9, protein 5

Poached Chicken with Rice

Why don't you try a healthy dash diet chicken dish today? Try this next suggestion!

Preparation time: 10 minutes
Cooking time: 40 minutes
Servings: 4

Ingredients:

- ½ tablespoon ginger, finely grated
- 3 garlic cloves, minced
- 1 tablespoon low sodium soy sauce
- 1 teaspoon black peppercorns
- 8 chicken legs
- 4 pak choi, halved
- Black pepper to the taste
- 2 bunches spring onions, chopped
- 3 tablespoons sesame oil
- Brown rice, already cooked for serving

Directions:

In a pan, mix ginger with half of the soy sauce, garlic, peppercorns and chicken. Add water to cover, season with black pepper to the taste, place on stove, bring to a boil over medium high heat, reduce temperature to low and simmer for 30 minutes. Heat up a pan with the oil over medium high heat, add onions, stir and cook for 1 minute. Take pan off heat, add soy sauce, stir well to make a relish and leave aside for now. Take chicken out of the pan and also leave aside to cool down on a plate. Add pak choi to chicken liquid, place on stove again on medium heat and cook for 4 minutes. Strain pak choi, discard solids and reserve cooking liquid. Discard skin and bones from chicken legs, shred meat and divide in bowls. Add rice on the side, pak choi, the relish you've made and some of the reserved cooking liquid. Enjoy!

Nutrition: calories 200, fat 2, fiber 4, carbs 7, protein 10

Hawaiian Chicken

It's intense, rich and flavored!

Preparation time: 4 hours and 10 minutes
Cooking time: 12 minutes
Servings: 4

Ingredients:

- 2 tablespoons tomato paste
- ¼ cup canned pineapple juice
- 2 tablespoons low sodium soy sauce
- 2 garlic cloves, minced
- 1 and ½ teaspoons ginger, grated
- 4 chicken breast halves, skinless and boneless
- Cooking spray
- Black pepper to the taste
- ¼ cup cilantro, chopped
- 2 cups brown rice, already cooked

Directions:

In a bowl, mix pineapple juice with tomato paste, soy sauce, garlic and ginger and stir well. Reserve ¼ cup of mix, transfer the rest to a zip-top bag, add chicken, seal bag, shake and keep in the fridge for 4 hours. Heat up a pan after you've sprayed some cooking oil in it over medium high heat, add marinated chicken and season with black pepper to the taste. Add the reserved marinade, stir and cook chicken for 6 minutes on each side. Add rice and cilantro, stir gently, take off heat and divide between plates. Enjoy!

Nutrition: calories 140, fat 1, fiber 4, carbs 9, protein 12

Easy Chicken Bites

These chicken bites are simply the best!

Preparation time: 10 minutes
Cooking time: 10 minutes
Servings: 4

Ingredients:

- 20 ounces canned pineapple slices
- A drizzle of olive oil
- 3 cups chicken thighs, boneless, skinless and cut into medium pieces
- 1 tablespoon smoked tea rub

Directions:

Heat up a pan over medium high heat, add pineapple slices, grill them for a few minutes on each side, transfer to a cutting board, cool them down and cut into medium cubes. Heat up a pan with a drizzle of oil over medium high heat, rub chicken pieces with smoked tea rub, place them in the pan and cook them for 10 minutes flipping from time to time. Arrange chicken cubes on a platter, add a pineapple piece on top and stick a toothpick in each. Serve right away!

Nutrition: calories 120, fat 3, fiber 1, carbs 5, protein 2

Impressive Chicken Salad

This is the perfect option for a quick meal!

Preparation time: 10 minutes
Cooking time: 30 minutes
Servings: 4

Ingredients:

- 1 whole chicken, chopped
- 8 black tea bags
- 4 scallions, chopped
- 2 celery ribs, chopped
- 1 cup mandarin orange, chopped
- ½ cup fat free yogurt
- 1 cup cashews, toasted and chopped
- Black pepper to the taste

Directions:

Put chicken pieces in a pot, add water to cover, also add tea bags, bring to a boil over medium heat and cook for 25 minutes until chicken is tender. Discard liquid and tea bags but reserve about 4 ounces. Transfer chicken to a cutting board, leave aside to cool down, discard bones, shred meat and put it in a bowl. Add celery, orange pieces, cashews, scallion and reserved liquid and toss everything. Add salt, pepper, mayo and yogurt, toss to coat well and keep in the fridge until you serve it. Enjoy!

Nutrition: calories 150, fat 3, fiber 3, carbs 7, protein 6

Incredible Chicken Chili

This is really spicy and extremely delicious!

Preparation time: 10 minutes
Cooking time: 1 hour and 10 minutes
Servings: 6

Ingredients:

- 1 cup white flour
- 1 tablespoon lemon juice
- Salt and black pepper to the taste
- 4 pounds chicken breast, skinless, boneless and cubed
- 4 ounces olive oil
- 4 ounces celery, chopped
- 1 tablespoon garlic, minced
- 8 ounces onion, chopped
- 5 ounces red bell pepper, chopped
- 7 ounces poblano pepper, chopped
- ¼ teaspoon cumin, ground
- 2 cups corn
- A pinch of cayenne pepper
- 1-quart chicken stock
- 1 teaspoon chili powder
- 16 ounces canned beans, drained
- ¼ cup cilantro, chopped

Directions:

Put flour in a bowl, add chicken pieces and toss well. Heat up a pan with the oil over medium high heat, add chicken, cook for 5 minutes on each side, transfer to a bowl and leave aside. Heat up the pan again over medium high heat, add onion, celery, garlic, bell pepper, poblano pepper and corn, stir and cook for 2 minutes more. Add stock, cumin, chili powder, beans, cayenne, cumin, salt, pepper, chicken pieces and lemon juice, stir, bring to a simmer, reduce heat to medium low, cover and cook for 1 hour. Add cilantro, stir, divide into bowls and serve right away! Enjoy!

Nutrition: calories 345, fat 2, fiber 3, carbs 9, protein 4

Savory Chicken Soup

This chicken noodle soup will warm up your heart!

Preparation time: 10 minutes
Cooking time: 15 minutes
Servings: 4

Ingredients:

- 4 cups chicken stock
- 1 teaspoon ginger, grated
- 1 tablespoon lemon juice
- 1 chicken breast, skinless, boneless, cooked and cut into medium pieces
- 2 garlic cloves, minced
- A pinch of sea salt
- Black pepper to the taste
- ½ cup egg noodles
- 2 carrots, chopped
- 1/3 cup parsley, chopped

Directions:

In a pot, mix chicken, stock, ginger, lemon juice, garlic, salt, pepper, carrots and noodles, stir, bring to a boil over medium high heat and simmer for 15 minutes. Add parsley, stir, ladle into bowls serve right away. Enjoy!

Nutrition: calories 145, fat 2, fiber 1, carbs 7, protein 21

Surprising Chicken and Peaches

You were looking for the combination! Make it today for your friends!

Preparation time: 10 minutes
Cooking time: 1 hour and 10 minutes
Servings: 4

Ingredients:

- 6 green tea and peach tea bags
- 1 whole chicken, cut into medium pieces
- ¾ cup water
- 1/3 cup honey
- Salt and black pepper to the taste
- ¼ cup olive oil
- 4 peaches, halved

Directions:

Put the water in a pot, bring to a simmer over medium heat, add tea bags, reduce heat to low and simmer for 10 minutes. Discard tea bags, add pepper and honey, whisk really well and leave aside. Rub chicken pieces with the oil, season with salt and pepper, place on preheated grill over medium high heat, brush with tea marinade, cover grill and cook for 15 minutes, Brush chicken with some more marinade, cook fro 15 minutes more and then flip again. Brush again with the tea marinade, cover and cook for 20 minutes more. Divide chicken pieces on plates and keep warm. Brush peaches with what's left of the tea and honey marinade, place them on your grill and cook for 4 minutes. Flip again and cook for 3 minutes more. Divide between plates next to chicken pieces and serve. Enjoy!

Nutrition: calories 500, fat 1, fiber 3, carbs 15, protein 10

Simple Glazed Chicken

This is really food for the soul!

Preparation time: 10 minutes
Cooking time: 1 hour and 10 minutes
Servings: 4

Ingredients:

- ½ cup apricot preserves
- ½ cup pineapple preserves
- 1 tablespoon low sodium soy sauce
- 1 onion, chopped
- ¼ teaspoon red pepper flakes
- 1 tablespoon vegetable oil
- Black pepper to the taste
- 6 chicken legs

Directions:

In a bowl, mix soy sauce, pepper flakes, apricot and pineapple preserves and whisk really well. Heat up a pan with the oil over medium high heat, add chicken pieces, cook them for 5 minutes on each side and transfer to a bowl. Spread onion on the bottom of a baking dish and add chicken pieces on top. Season with black pepper, drizzle the tea glaze on top, cover dish, introduce in the oven at 350 degrees F and bake for 30 minutes. Uncover dish and bake for 20 minutes more. Divide chicken on plates and keep warm. Pour cooking juices into a pan, heat up over medium high heat, cook until sauce is reduced and drizzle it over chicken pieces. Enjoy!

Nutrition: calories 198, fat 1, fiber 1, carbs 4, protein 19

Sesame and Ginger Steak

A hearty dish will suit even the most pretentious tastes!

Preparation time: 4 hours
Cooking time: 20 minutes
Servings: 6

Ingredients:

- 3 tablespoons peanut oil
- ¼ cup tamari
- 2 tablespoons mirin
- 1 and ½ teaspoons sesame oil
- 1 inch piece ginger, grated
- 2 garlic cloves, chopped
- 2 pounds beef meat, cubed
- 2 scallions, chopped
- 1 tablespoons sesame seeds, toasted

Directions:

In a bowl, mix peanut oil with tamari, ginger, garlic, mirin and sesame oil and stir very well. Add the meat, toss to coat, cover the bowl and keep in the fridge for 4 hours. Heat up your kitchen grill over medium temperature, add the meat and cook for 8 minutes turning from time to time. Transfer meat to a cutting board, leave aside to cool down for 10 minutes, thinly slice and arrange on a serving platter. Sprinkle scallions and sesame seeds on top and serve! Enjoy!

Nutrition: calories 150, fat 4, fiber 3, carbs 7, protein 12

Braised Beef Brisket

This is so delicious and rich!

Preparation time: 10 minutes
Cooking time: 7 hours and 15 minutes
Servings: 6

Ingredients:

- 1 pound sweet onion, chopped
- 4 pounds beef brisket
- 1 pound carrot, chopped
- 8 earl gray tea bags
- ½ pound celery, chopped
- A pinch of salt
- Black pepper to the taste
- 4 cups water

For the sauce:

- 16 ounces canned tomatoes, chopped
- ½ pound celery, chopped
- 1 ounce garlic, minced
- 4 ounces vegetable oil
- 1 pound sweet onion, chopped
- 1 cup palm sugar
- 8 earl gray tea bags
- 1 cup white vinegar

Directions:

Put the water in a pot, add 1 pound onion, 1 pound carrot, ½ pound celery, salt and pepper, stir and bring to a simmer over medium high heat. Add beef brisket and 8 tea bags, stir, cover, reduce heat to medium low and cook for 7 hours. Meanwhile, heat up a pan with the vegetable oil over medium high heat, add 1 pound onion, stir and sauté for 10 minutes. Add garlic, ½ pound celery, tomatoes, sugar, vinegar and 8 tea bags, stir, bring to a simmer, cook until veggies are done and discard tea bags at the end. Transfer beef brisket to a cutting board, leave aside to cool down, slice, divide between plates and serve with the sauce drizzled all over. Enjoy!

Nutrition: calories 400, fat 2, fiber 4, carbs 18, protein 3

Delicious Party Meatballs

Get ready to enjoy the best slow cooker dash diet party meatballs!

Preparation time: 10 minutes
Cooking time: 3 hours
Servings: 12

Ingredients:
- 1 tablespoon grill seasoning
- 1 tablespoon honey
- 1 egg, whisked
- ¼ cup low fat milk
- Black pepper to the taste
- 3 ounces low fat cheddar cheese, cubed
- 18 ounces low sodium BBQ sauce
- ½ cup bread crumbs
- 2 bacon slices, chopped
- 1 small yellow onion, chopped
- 1 pound beef, ground
- Cooking spray
- 24 dill pickle slices

Directions:

In a bowl, mix meat with onion, milk, egg, bread crumbs, bacon, black pepper, honey and grill seasoning, stir very well and shape 24 balls. Stick a cheese cube in each meatball, seal well, spray your slow cooker with cooking oil and arrange meatballs on it. Add BBQ sauce to them, spread well, cover slow cooker and cook on Low for 3 hours. Place a pickle slice in each meatball, secure with toothpicks, arrange on a platter serve. Enjoy!

Nutrition: calories 200, fat 2, fiber 6, carbs 20, protein 5

Superb Beef Stew

Everyone will say that this is the best and most delicious dash diet beef stews ever!

Preparation time: 10 minutes
Cooking time: 7 hours
Servings: 6

Ingredients:
- 32 ounces low sodium beef stock
- 2 tablespoons low sodium Worcestershire sauce
- 3 garlic cloves, minced
- 6 ounces tomato paste
- 2 cups baby carrots
- 1 yellow onion, chopped
- 2 celery ribs, chopped
- Black pepper to the taste
- 2 pounds beef stew meat, cubed
- 1 cup peas
- 1 tablespoon parsley, dried
- 1 teaspoon oregano, dried
- 1 cup corn
- ¼ cup water
- ¼ cup white flour

Directions:

In your slow cooker, mix beef with carrots, onion, celery, salt, pepper, stock, garlic, oregano, parsley, peas, corn, Worcestershire sauce and tomato paste, stir, cover and cook on High for 6 hours and 30 minutes. In a bowl, mix flour with water, stir well and pour into the stew. Stir well and cook on High for 30 minutes more. Divide into bowls and serve. Enjoy!

Nutrition: calories 200, fat 2, fiber 6, carbs 20, protein 5

Beef Stroganoff

This is one recipe we are sure you will want to learn how to make!

Preparation time: 10 minutes
Cooking time: 20 minutes
Servings: 4

Ingredients:

- 24 ounces beef tenderloin
- A pinch of sea salt
- Black pepper to the taste
- ¼ cup olive oil
- 2 tablespoons olive oil
- 2 cups button mushrooms, chopped
- ½ cup low sodium veggie stock
- 2 tablespoons flour
- 1/3 cup fat free milk
- 2/3 cup fat free yogurt
- 1 tablespoon mustard
- A few springs parsley, chopped

Directions:

Heat up a pan with 1 tablespoon oil over medium high heat, add steaks, season with salt and pepper, cook for 4 minutes, flip and cook for 4 more minutes, take off heat and transfer to a plate. Add 1 more tablespoon oil to the pan, add mushrooms, stir, cook for 4 minutes and transfer to a bowl. Heat up another pan with the rest of the oil over low heat, add flour and stir very well. Add stock, mustard, yogurt, black pepper and milk, stir and cook until everything thickens. Divide meat on plates, add mushrooms and top with the sauce. Serve hot! Enjoy!

Nutrition: calories 200, fat 2, fiber 4, carbs 20, protein 7

Simple Zucchini and Pork Stir Fry

You don't need to be an expert in the kitchen to make this stir fry!

Preparation time: 10 minutes
Cooking time: 10 minutes
Servings: 3

Ingredients:

- 1 tablespoon rice wine
- 3.5 ounces pork tenderloin, sliced
- Black pepper to the taste
- 1 tablespoon cornstarch
- 1 teaspoon ginger, grated
- 2 tablespoons peanut oil
- 3 garlic cloves, minced
- 2 dried chili peppers, chopped
- 2 teaspoons low sodium soy sauce
- 1 zucchini, sliced

Directions:

In a bowl, mix pork with rice wine, pepper, cornstarch and ginger, toss to coat and leave aside for 15 minutes. Heat up a pan with half of the oil over medium high heat, add pork, stir, cook for 1 minutes, transfer to a plate and leave aside. Heat up the pan with the rest of the oil over medium heat, add chili peppers, garlic and zucchini pieces, stir and cook for 1 minute. Return pork to pan, add soy sauce, some salt and pepper, stir and cook for 6 minutes. Divide between plates and serve. Enjoy!

Nutrition: calories 150, fat 4, fiber 5, carbs 9, protein 5

Pork Chops with Apples And Onions

Gather your loved ones and enjoy this perfect, healthy dish!

Preparation time: 10 minutes
Cooking time: 20 minutes
Servings: 4

Ingredients:

- 1 and ½ cups pearl onions
- 2 and ½ teaspoons canola oil
- 2 cups apple, cut into wedges
- A pinch of sea salt
- Black pepper to the taste
- 2 teaspoons thyme, chopped
- 4 medium pork loin chops, bone-in
- 1 teaspoon cider vinegar
- ½ teaspoon white flour
- ½ cup low sodium chicken stock

Directions:

Heat up a pan with 1 teaspoon oil over medium high heat, pat dry pearl onions, add to pan and cook for 2 minutes. Add apple, stir, introduce pan in the oven at 400 degrees F and bake for 10 minutes. Take out of the oven, add salt, pepper and thyme and stir gently. Heat up another pan with 1 and ½ teaspoon oil over medium high heat, add pork after you've seasoned it with salt and pepper to the taste, cook for 3 minutes on each side, remove from pan and keep warm. Put stock in a pot, add flour, stir well, heat up, bring to a boil and cook for 1 minutes. Add vinegar and the rest of the butter, stir and take off heat. Arrange pork chops on serving plates, add apple and onion mix on the side and serve with the sauce you've just made. Enjoy!

Nutrition: calories 240, fat 10, fiber 2, carbs 10, protein 24

Baby Back Ribs and Tasty Salad

It's a fulfilling dinner idea for you and your loved ones!

Preparation time: 1 hour and 10 minutes
Cooking time: 1 hour
Servings: 6

Ingredients:

- 12 green tea bags, strings removed
- Salt and black pepper to the taste
- 26 pork back ribs
- 1 onion, julienned
- 3 carrots, chopped
- 6 celery ribs, chopped
- 1 Jicama, roughly chopped
- 2 green apples, chopped
- 4 scallions, chopped
- ½ cup rice wine vinegar
- 1 green tea and lemon tea bag
- 1 cup olive oil

Directions:

In a pot, mix ribs with salt, pepper, half of the carrot, onion, half of the celery and 8 tea bags, stir, bring to a simmer over medium heat, cover and cook for 1 hour. Meanwhile, in a bowl, mix vinegar with green tea and lemon tea bag, stir, leave aside for 1 hour and discard tea bags. In a bowl, mix apple with the rest of the celery ribs, the rest of the carrot, Jicama, scallions and oil and toss to coat. Add vinaigrette and toss to coat. Divide ribs on plates and return cooking liquid to medium heat. Bring to a simmer, add the rest of the tea bags, cook for 10 minutes and discard them. Drizzle this over ribs and serve with the salad on the side. Enjoy!

Nutrition: calories 400, fat 7, fiber 3, carbs 20, protein 4

Simple Pork Soup

Don't hesitate to try this soup! It's easy to make and it's delicious!

Preparation time: 10 minutes
Cooking time: 20 minutes
Servings: 3

Ingredients:

- ½ pounds pork meat, thinly sliced
- 1 yellow onion, chopped
- 3 teaspoons low sodium fish sauce
- 1 big eggplant, chopped
- 4 tomatoes, chopped
- 4 cups water
- 1 bunch red Shiso, stems removed

Directions:

Heat up a pot over medium high heat, add onions, stir and cook for 3-4 minutes. Add pork, stir and cook until it browns.Add the water, stir and bring to a boil. Add tomatoes and eggplants, stir, bring to a boil, reduce heat to medium and simmer for 15 minutes. Add shiso leaves and fish sauce, stir well, pour into soup bowls and serve. Enjoy!

Nutrition: calories 140, fat 3, fiber 5, carbs 10, protein 5

Thai Steak Delight

This is really a delightful meal for you to share with your family tonight!

Preparation time: 1 hour and 10 minutes
Cooking time: 12 minutes
Servings: 4

Ingredients:

- 1 pound steak
- 1 tablespoon vegetable oil
- 2 tablespoons low sodium soy sauce
- ½ teaspoon ginger, grated
- 1 garlic cloves, minced
- 16 ounces salad greens
- 1 carrot, grated
- ½ bunch green onions, chopped

For the dressing:

- 2 tablespoons sugar
- ¼ cup white vinegar
- ¾ teaspoon ginger, grated
- 1 tablespoon vegetable oil
- A pinch of salt

Directions:

In a bowl, mix steak with soy sauce, 1 tablespoon oil, garlic and ½ teaspoon ginger, toss well, cover and keep in the fridge for 1 hour. Heat up your grill over medium high heat, add steak, cook for 6 minutes, flip, cook for 6 more minutes, transfer to a cutting board, leave aside to cool down a bit and slice. Heat up a pan over medium high heat, add vinegar, sugar, 1 tablespoon oil, a pinch of salt and ¾ teaspoon ginger, stir well and cook until sugar dissolves. Take off heat and leave aside to cool down. In a salad bowl, combine mixed salad greens with carrot and onions. Add steak slices, the salad dressing, toss gently and serve. Enjoy!

Nutrition: calories 150, fat 2, fiber 5, carbs 8, protein 12

Spicy Beef Stir Fry

This is a spicy dinner idea! Try it!

Preparation time: 10 minutes
Cooking time: 7 minutes
Servings: 4

Ingredients:

- 2 teaspoons ginger, grated
- 3 cups mixed veggies (carrots, celery)
- 4 teaspoons canola oil
- 8 ounces beef sirloin, cut into thin strips
- 1 cup edamame
- 3 tablespoons hoisin sauce
- 1 teaspoon red chili paste
- 2 tablespoons rice vinegar
- 8 ounces long grain rice, already cooked

Directions:

Heat up a pan with half of the oil over medium high heat, add ginger, stir and cook for 15 minutes. Add mixed veggies, stir, cook for 4 minutes and transfer to a bowl. Heat up the pan with the rest of the oil over medium high heat, add edamame and beef, stir and cook for 2 minutes. Return veggies to the pan, stir and cook for 1 minute more. Meanwhile, in a bowl, mix chili paste with vinegar and hoisin sauce and stir really well. Add this to the pan with the beef, stir well, take off heat and divide between plates. Add rice on the side and serve. Enjoy!

Nutrition: calories 150, fat 2, fiber 3, carbs 10, protein 6

Special Steak Salad

This salad is served with a special dressing on top! It's heavenly!

Preparation time: 10 minutes
Cooking time: 4 minutes
Servings: 4

Ingredients:

- 8 cups mixed salad greens
- 2 carrots, cut into thin matchsticks
- 1 yellow bell pepper, cut into thin strips
- 1 cup cherry tomatoes, halved
- 8 ounces beef sirloin cut into thin strips
- Cooking spray
- ¼ cup basil, chopped

For the salad dressing:
- ½ cup low fat sour cream
- ½ cup low fat buttermilk
- 2 garlic cloves, minced
- White pepper to the taste
- A pinch of salt
- 2 teaspoons lemon juice
- ¼ cup chives, chopped
- 1 and ½ teaspoon dill, chopped
- A splash of Tabasco sauce

Directions:

In a bowl, mix buttermilk with sour cream, salt, pepper, garlic, chives, dill, lemon juice and Tabasco sauce, stir really well and leave aside for now. Heat up a pan with cooking spray over medium high heat, add beef strips, cook for 4 minutes and transfer to a bowl. Add greens, carrots, bell pepper and cherry tomatoes and toss gently. Add salad dressing, toss to coat and serve with basil sprinkled on top. Enjoy!

Nutrition: calories 160, fat 2, fiber 5, carbs 12, protein 4

Delicious Lamb

This can be served on a special occasion! No one with notice that it's a diet dish!

Preparation time: 4 hours and 10 minutes
Cooking time: 50 minutes
Servings: 8

Ingredients:

- 2 pounds lamb rib roasts
- 1 cup red wine
- 1 teaspoon nutmeg, ground
- 2 garlic cloves, minced
- 3 tablespoons olive oil
- 1 tablespoon ghee
- 2 cups bread crumbs
- 1 tablespoons rosemary, chopped
- 1 tablespoon lavender, dried
- A pinch of sea salt
- Black pepper to the taste

Directions:

In a bowl, mix lamb ribs with wine, 1 garlic clove and nutmeg, cover and keep in the fridge for 4 hours. Heat up a pan with 1 tablespoon oil and the ghee over medium heat, add the rest of the garlic and rosemary, stir and cook for 1 minute. Add breadcrumbs, stir and cook for 3 minutes. Take off heat, add a pinch of salt, black pepper, cranberries and lavender and stir well. Add the rest of the oil and stir really well. Transfer lamb ribs to a baking dish, press breadcrumbs mix on it, add marinade to the dish as well, introduce in the oven at 450 degrees F and roast for 30 minutes. Leave lamb ribs to cool down a bit before serving them. Enjoy!

Nutrition: calories 179, fat 1, fiber 5, carbs 20, protein 6

Wonderful Beef

It's so yummy and easy to make!

Preparation time: 10 minutes
Cooking time: 15 minutes
Servings: 4

Ingredients:

- 1 cup green onion, sliced
- 1 cup low sodium soy sauce
- ½ cup water
- ½ cup dry sherry
- ¼ cup brown sugar
- ¼ cup sesame seeds
- 5 garlic cloves, minced
- Black pepper to the taste
- 1 pound lean beef, sliced
- Already cooked brown rice for serving
- Chopped green onions for serving

Directions:

In a bowl, mix onion with soy sauce, water, sugar, sherry, garlic, sesame seeds and pepper and stir well. Place meat in a large dish, pour marinade over, cover and leave aside for 10 minutes. Drain meat, place on preheated kitchen grill over medium high heat and cook for 15 minutes flipping once. Divide on plate sand serve with brown rice on the side and green onions sprinkled on top. Enjoy!

Nutrition: calories 239, fat 3, fiber 5, carbs 13, protein 6

Simple Thai Pork

This quick dish tastes divine!

Preparation time: 10 minutes
Cooking time: 10 minutes
Servings: 4

Ingredients:
- 1 cup jasmine rice, already cooked
- 1 teaspoon olive oil
- 2 teaspoons low sodium soy sauce
- ½ teaspoon ginger, grated
- 3 garlic cloves, minced
- ½ pound pork tenderloin, cut into strips
- Juice from 1 lime
- ¼ cup cilantro, chopped
- 1 pound papaya, peeled and cubed

Directions:

Heat up a large pan with the oil over medium high heat, add pork, stir and cook for 3 minutes. Add soy sauce, garlic and ginger, stir and cook for 5 more minutes. Remove pan from heat, add lime juice, papaya and cilantro and toss to coat. Divide between plates and serve with the rice on the side. Enjoy!

Nutrition: calories 200, fat 3, fiber 2, carbs 8, protein 10

Lamb Meatballs and Mint Sauce

Oh my God! What a delicious dash diet combination!

Preparation time: 10 minutes
Cooking time: 15 minutes
Servings: 24

Ingredients:
- 10 ounces lamb meat, ground
- 2 teaspoons garlic, minced
- 2 teaspoons ginger, grated
- 2 teaspoons chili peppers, minced
- 2 tablespoons coriander, chopped
- 2 tablespoons low sodium fish sauce
- 1 egg
- 1 cup breadcrumbs
- Black pepper to the taste
- Vegetable oil for frying
- 2 tablespoons honey

For the mint sauce:
- 1 teaspoon ginger, grated
- 4 tablespoons rice wine
- 2 tablespoons low sodium soy sauce
- 2 tablespoons mint, chopped
- 1 teaspoon sugar
- Back pepper to the taste

Directions:

In a bowl, mix lamb meat with 2 teaspoons ginger, garlic, chili, coriander, fish sauce, egg, black pepper to the taste and breadcrumbs and stir well. Shape meatballs out of this mix and place them all on a working surface. Heat up a large pan with the oil over medium high heat, add meatballs and cook them for 4 minutes on each side. Transfer to paper towels, drain grease, drizzle the honey over them and arrange on a platter. Meanwhile, in a bowl, mix 1 teaspoon ginger with rice vinegar, soy sauce, chopped mint, sugar and pepper to the taste. Transfer sauce to small bowls serve with your lamb meatballs. Enjoy!

Nutrition: calories 279, fat 2, fiber 4, carbs 10, protein 10

Exotic Pork Soup

You should try this special and exotic soup today!

Preparation time: 25 minutes
Cooking time: 10 minutes
Servings: 2

Ingredients:

- 1/8 pound pork loin, sliced
- 1 tablespoon rice wine
- Black pepper to the taste
- 1 cup sour Kimchi, chopped and juice reserved
- 1 green onion, sliced
- ¼ cup mushrooms, chopped
- 3 tablespoons Anaheim green chili peppers, sliced
- 1 cup tofu, cubed
- 1 and ½ cup water
- 1 tablespoon vegetable oil
- 4 teaspoons chili flakes
- 2 teaspoons chili paste
- 4 teaspoons low sodium soy sauce
- ½ teaspoon garlic, minced

Directions:

In a bowl, mix pork meat with rice wine and some black pepper and leave aside for 15 minutes. Heat up a big pan with the oil over medium high heat, add Kimchi, cook for 5 minutes stirring often, take off heat and transfer to a bowl. Meanwhile, in another bowl, mix chili flakes with chili paste, soy sauce, garlic and black pepper. Add kimchi, green onion, green chili peppers and mushrooms. Transfer everything in a pot, add the water and the kimchi juice, stir and bring to a boil over medium high heat. Add meat, stir and simmer everything for 5 minutes. Reduce heat to low, add tofu, stir gently, ladle into bowls and serve. Enjoy!

Nutrition: calories 130, fat 1, fiber 5, carbs 10, protein 2

Pork Medallions and Delicious Slaw

This is such a tasty dash diet meal! It's really impressive!

Preparation time: 40 minutes
Cooking time: 5 minutes
Servings: 6
Ingredients:

- 2 medium pork tenderloins, fat removed and cut into medium size medallions
- ¼ cup rice vinegar
- 1/3 cup low sodium soy sauce
- 2 garlic cloves, minced
- 3 tablespoons brown sugar
- 1 and ½ tablespoons ginger, grated
- 1 tablespoon sesame oil
- 3 teaspoons Sriracha chili sauce
- 6 cups napa cabbage, shredded
- 2 carrots, grated
- 4 scallions, chopped
- 5 tablespoons canola oil
- Black pepper to the taste

Directions:

In a small bowl, mix soy sauce with 2 tablespoons brown sugar, 2 tablespoons rice vinegar, garlic, ½ tablespoon sesame oil, ginger and 2 teaspoons chili sauce and stir well. Mix half of this combination with pork medallions in a separate bowl and leave the rest aside. Leave the meat to marinate for 25 minutes. Meanwhile, in another bowl, mix cabbage with carrot and half of the scallions. Add 1 tablespoon canola oil, black pepper to the taste, 2 tablespoons rice vinegar, ½ tablespoon sesame oil, 1 tablespoon brown sugar and 1 teaspoon chili sauce, stir and leave aside. Heat up a pan with 2 tablespoons canola oil over medium high heat , add half of the pork medallions, cook for 2 minutes, flip, cook for 2 minutes more and transfer to a plate. Clean up the pan, add the other 2 tablespoons of canola oil, heat up again over medium high heat, add the rest of the pork medallions and cook them as well. Divide slaw on plates, add medallions on top and drizzle the reserved soy and ginger sauce on top. Sprinkle the rest of the scallions at the end and serve right away! Enjoy!

Nutrition: calories 200, fat 3, fiber 3, carbs 10, protein 5

Flavored Steak

Try this dash diet dish and enjoy a very special texture and flavor!

Preparation time: 20 minutes
Cooking time: 6 minutes
Servings: 4

Ingredients:

- 1 pound beef steaks, sliced
- 2 tablespoons brown sugar
- 3 tablespoons low sodium soy sauce
- 2 teaspoons sake
- 4 garlic cloves, minced
- 5 scallions, chopped
- 2 teaspoons ginger, grated
- 2 teaspoons sesame oil
- 2 teaspoons vegetable oil
- Black pepper to the taste

Directions:

In a bowl, mix steaks with sugar with soy sauce, sake, scallions, ginger, garlic and sesame oil, toss well and leave aside for 20 minutes. Heat up a pan with the vegetable oil over medium high heat, add steaks, season with black pepper to the taste and cook for 3 minutes on each side. Transfer to a working surface, leave aside to cool down for a couple of minutes, cut into thin strips and serve with a side salad on the side. Enjoy!

Nutrition: calories 150, fat 2, fiber 4, carbs 8, protein 4

Thai Style Beef

This time try something really delicious today!

Preparation time: 40 minutes
Cooking time: 10 minutes
Servings: 8

Ingredients:

- 1 pound beef steak, sliced
- ½ cup red curry paste
- 1 cup coconut milk
- 1 tablespoon brown sugar
- 2 tablespoons low sodium fish sauce
- 1 teaspoon turmeric
- Cooking spray
- 2 tablespoons coconut cream
- 1 tablespoon red curry paste
- 1 cup low sodium chicken stock
- 1 tablespoon peanut butter
- 1 tablespoon lime juice

Directions:

In a bowl, mix steak with ½ cup red curry paste, ½ cup coconut milk, 1 tablespoon sugar, 1 tablespoon fish sauce and 1 teaspoon turmeric, toss to coat and keep in the fridge for 30 minutes. Heat up your grill, thread the beef on skewers, spray them with some cooking oil and cook them for about 3-4 minutes. Transfer to a serving plate and leave covered for now. Meanwhile, heat up a small pan at a medium temperature and add the coconut cream in it. Leave aside for about 2 minutes, add 1 tablespoon red curry paste and ½ cup coconut milk and stir very well. Add chicken stock, peanut butter, 1 tablespoon fish sauce and lime juice, stir and boil for about 10 minutes over low heat. Divide beef between plates and serve with the peanut sauce drizzled all over. Enjoy!

Nutrition: calories 150, fat 3, fiber 3, carbs 10, protein 3

Pork Medallions and Delicious Pear Sauce

The combination is so much better that you can imagine it!

Preparation time: 10 minutes
Cooking time: 10 minutes
Servings: 4

Ingredients:

- 1 medium pork tenderloin, sliced
- 1 teaspoons rosemary, chopped
- ¼ teaspoon thyme, dried
- A pinch of sea salt
- Black pepper to the taste
- 2 pears, peeled and chopped
- 1 tablespoon olive oil
- 2 tablespoons red cherries, dried and halved
- ¼ cup maple syrup
- 2 tablespoons white wine

Directions:

In a bowl, mix rosemary with thyme, salt, pepper and stir. Add meat and toss to coat. Heat up a pan with the oil over medium high heat, add meat slices, cook them for 3 minutes, flip, cook them for 3 minutes more and transfer to a plate. Heat up the same pan over medium heat, add pears, cherries, wine and maple syrup, stir, bring to a boil and simmer for 3 minutes. Return meat to the pan, stir again, divide everything between plates and serve. Enjoy!

Nutrition: calories 300, fat 3, fiber 4, carbs 17, protein 4

Incredible Pork Roast

This dash diet pork roast is perfect for the holidays!

Preparation time: 10 minutes
Cooking time: 2 hours and 10 minutes
Servings: 8

Ingredients:

- 1 pork loin roast
- 1 tablespoon maple syrup
- 2 tablespoons mustard
- 1 teaspoon orange peel, grated
- 2 teaspoons sage, dried
- A pinch of sea salt
- Black pepper to the taste
- 20 small new potatoes, peeled
- 16 ounces baby carrots
- 1 tablespoon olive oil

Directions:

In a bowl, mix mustard with maple syrup, salt, pepper, orange peel and sage and stir. Spread this over pork roast, place in a roasting pan, introduce in the oven at 325 degrees F and roast for 45 minutes. Put some water in a pot, bring to a boil over medium high heat, add potatoes and cook for 5 minutes. Add carrots, stir and cook for 5 minutes more. Drain veggies, transfer to a bowl, add black pepper and the oil and toss to coat. Place them in the roasting pan with the roast, introduce in the oven again and roast for 45 minutes more. Leave everything to cool down, divide roast and veggies between plates and serve warm. Enjoy!

Nutrition: calories 270, fat 3, fiber 4, carbs 19, protein 5

Amazing Beef Kabobs

These are what you need for a summer gathering!

Preparation time: 10 minutes
Cooking time: 12 minutes
Servings: 4

Ingredients:

- 12 ounces beef steak, cubed
- 1 tablespoon vegetable oil
- 2 tablespoons red wine vinegar
- 1 tablespoon Jamaican seasoning
- 2 plantains, peeled and cut into chunks
- 1 red onion, cut into wedges
- Mixed salad greens for salad

Directions:

In a bowl, mix Jamaica seasoning with vinegar and oil and stir. Add meat, plantain and onion pieces and toss to coat. Thread everything on skewers, brush them with the remaining marinade, place skewers on preheated grill over medium high heat, cook for 7 minutes, flip and cook for 7 minutes more. Divide between plates and serve with mixed salad greens on the side. Enjoy!

Nutrition: calories 190, fat 3, fiber 4, carbs 8, protein 5

Herbed Sirloin Steak

It's really flavored! Trust us!

Preparation time: 10 minutes
Cooking time: 12 minutes
Servings: 6

Ingredients:

- 2 tablespoons catsup
- 1 and ½ teaspoons rosemary, chopped
- Black pepper to the taste
- 1and ½ teaspoons basil, chopped
- A pinch of garlic powder
- 1 and ½ pounds beef sirloin, sliced
- A pinch of cardamom, ground
- Grilled sweet peppers for serving

Directions:

In a bowl, mix catsup with rosemary, black pepper, basil, garlic powder and cardamom and stir. Add beef, toss to coat well, place on preheated grill over medium high heat and cook for 6 minutes on each side. Divide between plates and serve with grilled sweet peppers on the side. Enjoy!

Nutrition: calories 130, fat 2, fiber 5, carbs 8, protein 6

Delicious Steak and Tasty Corn Salsa

The combination is just right!

Preparation time: 12 hours and 10 minutes
Cooking time: 20 minutes
Servings: 6

Ingredients:

- 8 ounces canned corn, drained
- 1 tomato, chopped
- ¾ cup bottled Salsa Verde
- 1 and ½ pounds beef steak, sliced
- ¾ cup bottled Italian salad dressing
- 1 teaspoon cumin, ground
- 1 tablespoon Worcestershire sauce
- Black pepper to the taste

Directions:

In a bowl, mix salsa Verde with tomato can corn, stir, cover and keep in the fridge fro 6 hours. Meanwhile, in another bowl, mix steak with Italian salad dressing, Worcestershire sauce, cumin and black pepper, toss to coat and also keep in the fridge for 6 hours. Heat up your grill over medium high heat, add steaks, cook for 10 minutes on each side and divide between plates. Add corn salsa on the side and serve. Enjoy!

Nutrition: calories 200, fat 1, fiber 4, carbs 20, protein 5

Dash Diet Dessert Recipes

Carrot Cake

It looks so beautiful and it tastes wonderful!

Preparation time: 3 hours and 10 minutes
Cooking time: 0 minutes
Servings: 6

Ingredients:
For the cashew frosting:
- 2 tablespoons lemon juice
- 2 cups cashews, soaked for a couple of hours and drained
- 2 tablespoons coconut oil, melted
- 1/3 cup maple syrup
- Water

For the cake:
- 1 cup pineapple, dried and chopped
- 2 carrots, chopped
- 1 and ½ cups whole wheat flour
- 1 cup dates, pitted and chopped
- ½ cup dry coconut flakes
- ½ teaspoon cinnamon, ground

Directions:
In your blender, mix cashews with lemon juice, coconut oil, maple syrup and some apple, pulse very well, transfer to a bowl and leave aside for now. Put carrots in your food processor and pulse them a few times. Add flour, dates, pineapple, coconut and cinnamon and pulse very well again. Pour half of this mix into a springform pan and spread evenly. Add 1/3 of the frosting and also spread. Add the rest of the cake mix and the rest of the frosting. Introduce in the freezer and keep there before serving. Enjoy!

Nutrition: calories 140, fat 2, fiber 4, carbs 7, protein 4

Simple Mandarin Cake

It's an excellent option for dessert!

Preparation time: 2 hours and 10 minutes
Cooking time: 0 minutes
Yield: 6

Ingredients:
- 3 carrots, grated
- 1/3 cup dates, pitted and chopped
- 4 mandarins, peeled and roughly chopped
- A handful walnuts, soaked in water for 5 hours and drained
- 8 tablespoons coconut oil
- 1 cup cashews, soaked for 2 hours and drained
- Juice from 2 lemons
- 2 tablespoons stevia
- Some water
- A pinch of turmeric

Directions:
In your food processor, mix carrots with dates, walnuts, mandarins and half of the coconut oil, blend very well and transfer to a bowl. Clean your food processor, add cashews with lemon juice, stevia, water and a pinch of turmeric and blend very well. Add the rest of the oil and blend again. Pour the carrot mix in a cake form and spread it well. Add the lemon cream and spread well again. Keep in the fridge for a few hours before you cut and serve it. Enjoy!

Nutrition: calories 130, fat 2, fiber 3, carbs 5, protein 1

Carrot Cupcakes

We adore these cupcakes!

Preparation time: 1 hour and 10 minutes
Cooking time: 0 minutes
Servings: 6

Ingredients:

- 1 cup almonds
- 2 cups carrot pulp
- 1 cup dates, chopped
- ½ teaspoon ginger, grated
- 1 teaspoon cinnamon powder
- A pinch of nutmeg
- ¾ cup raisins
- A pinch of salt

For the frosting:

- 1 cup cashews, soaked for 1 hour and drained
- A pinch of salt
- A splash of water
- 1 teaspoon lemon juice
- 6 dates, pitted, soaked for 1 hour and drained

Directions:

In your food processor, mix 1 cup walnuts with 1 cup dates, carrot pulp, 1 teaspoon cinnamon, ginger, a pinch of nutmeg, a pinch of salt and the raisins and blend very well. Divide this between cupcakes tins and push it well. Clean your food processor, add 1 cup cashews, 6 dates, a pinch of salt, a splash of water and the lemon juice and blend these as well. Divide the frosting on the cupcakes, introduce them in the fridge and keep there for 1 hour. Enjoy!

Nutrition: calories 150, fat 2, fiber 2, carbs 3, protein 1

Green Tea Sorbet

Here's another delicious and classic dash diet dessert!

Preparation time: 6 hours and 5 minutes
Cooking time: 0 minutes
Servings: 4

Ingredients:

- 4 tablespoons canned coconut milk
- 1 cup fat free coconut cream
- 3 tablespoons hot water
- 4 and ½ teaspoons green tea powder

Directions:

In a bowl, mix green tea powder with hot water, stir well and leave aside until it's cold. Add milk and cream, stir again well, transfer to a container and freeze for 6 hours before serving. Enjoy!

Nutrition: calories 200, fat 2, fiber 5, carbs 10, protein 4

Spring Smoothie Bowl

It's easy and so delicious!

Preparation time: 10 minutes
Cooking time: 0 minutes
Servings: 1

Ingredients:

- ½ cup coconut water
- 1 and ½ cup avocado, pitted, peeled and chopped
- 1 big banana, peeled and chopped
- 2 tablespoons green tea powder
- 2 teaspoons lime zest
- 1 tablespoon palm sugar
- 1 mango, thinly sliced for serving

Directions:

In your blender, mix water with banana, avocado, green tea powder and lime zest and pulse well. Add palm sugar and pulse again well. Transfer to a bowl, top with sliced mango and serve. Enjoy!

Nutrition: calories 137, fat 2, fiber 10, carbs 20, protein 5

Simple Matcha Doughnuts

These are surprisingly delicious!

Preparation time: 10 minutes
Cooking time: 10 minutes
Servings: 8

Ingredients:

- ¼ cup brown sugar
- 1 cup whole wheat flour
- 1 teaspoon baking powder
- 2 tablespoons matcha powder
- ½ teaspoon vanilla extract
- ½ cup low fat buttermilk
- 1 egg, whisked
- ½ teaspoon vanilla extract
- 1 tablespoon ghee, melted
- Cooking spray

Directions:

Spray a doughnut pan with cooking spray and leave aside. In a bowl, mix flour with matcha powder, sugar and baking powder and whisk well. Add buttermilk, vanilla extract, egg and butter and stir using your mixer. Divide into doughnut cavities, introduce in the oven at 400 degrees F and bake for 10 minutes. Leave doughnuts to cool down before serving them. Enjoy!

Nutrition: calories 200, fat 2, fiber 3, carbs 7, protein 4

Figs Dessert

This is super easy to make it home!

Preparation time: 6 minutes
Cooking time: 4 minutes
Servings: 3

Ingredients:
- 2 tablespoons coconut butter
- 12 figs, halved
- ¼ cup palm sugar
- 1 cup almonds blanched and toasted

Directions:
Put butter in a pot over high heat and melt it. Add figs, sugar, stir and cook for 4 minutes. Add almonds, toss to coat, transfer to bowls and serve! Enjoy!

Nutrition: calories 220, fat 2, fiber 1, carbs 2, protein 9

Chocolate Jelly

It's so delicious and easy to make!

Preparation time: 1 hour and 10 minutes
Cooking time: 20 minutes
Servings: 4

Ingredients:
- 3 ounces dark and unsweetened chocolate
- 1 cup warm water
- 1 tablespoon vanilla extract
- 2 cups low fat milk
- 3 tablespoons brown sugar
- 2 tablespoons gelatin

Directions:
In a bowl, mix warm water with gelatin, stir well and leave aside for 1 hour. Put this in a pot and heat up over medium heat. In another pot, mix milk with sugar and chocolate, stir and bring to a boil over medium heat. Add gelatin and vanilla, stir, transfer to molds and leave aside to completely cool down before serving! Enjoy!

Nutrition: calories 100, fat 1, fiber 1, carbs 2, protein 2

Delicious Energy Bars

This is so good! Try it soon!

Preparation time: 10 minutes
Cooking time: 30 minutes
Servings: 6

Ingredients:
- 1 pound sunflower seeds mixed with walnuts, almonds and peanuts, chopped
- 2 cups honey
- 6 tablespoons sugar

Directions:
Spread nuts on a baking sheet, introduce in the oven at 350 degrees F and roast them for 10 minutes. Meanwhile, in a pan, mix honey with sugar, stir and bring to a boil over medium heat. Take nuts out of the oven, add them to the pan, stir and cook for 15 minutes more. Pour this mix into a pan brushed with water, spread evenly and leave aside to cool down. Turn pan upside down, cut rectangles and serve them cold. Enjoy!

Nutrition: calories 100, fat 2, fiber 3, carbs 7, protein 1

Mexican Tomato Dessert

Can you gather all the ingredients and make this dash diet dessert today?

Preparation time: 10 minutes
Cooking time: 40 minutes
Servings: 4

Ingredients:

- 5 pounds tomatoes, blanched for a few seconds and peeled
- 3 cups coconut sugar
- 3 cups water
- ½ teaspoon cinnamon powder
- 2 cinnamon sticks
- 2 teaspoons vanilla
- ½ teaspoon cloves, ground

Method:

Bring the water to a boil in a pot over medium heat, add tomatoes and boil them for 30 minutes. Add cinnamon sticks, cinnamon, sugar, vanilla and cloves and simmer until sugar dissolves. Take off heat, discard cinnamon stick, leave aside to cool down, divide into bowls and serve! Enjoy!

Nutrition: calories 150, fat 1, fiber 1, carbs 5, protein 4

Special Tomato Cake

Try something really special today!

Preparation time: 10 minutes
Cooking time: 35 minutes
Servings: 6

Ingredients:

- 1 and ½ cups whole wheat flour
- 1 teaspoon cinnamon, ground
- 1 teaspoon baking soda
- 1 teaspoon baking powder
- ¾ cup brown sugar
- 1 cup tomatoes, blanched, deseeded, peeled and chopped
- ½ cup olive oil
- 2 tablespoons apple cider vinegar

Directions:

In a bowl, mix flour with sugar, cinnamon, baking powder and soda and stir well. In another bowl, mix tomatoes with oil and cider vinegar and also stir very well. Combine the 2 mixtures, stir, pour everything into a greased round baking pan, introduce in the oven at 350 degrees F and bake for 35 minutes. Leave the cake to cool down before slicing and serving it. Enjoy!

Nutrition: calories 100, fat 2, fiber 1, carbs 1, protein 3

Maple Cupcakes

They're so delicious!

Preparation time: 10 minutes
Cooking time: 30 minutes
Servings: 4

Ingredients:

- 4 tablespoons coconut butter
- 4 eggs
- ½ cup applesauce
- 2 teaspoons cinnamon
- 1 teaspoon vanilla extract
- ½ apple, cored, peeled and sliced
- 4 teaspoons maple syrup
- ¾ cup almond flour
- ½ teaspoon baking powder
- Cinnamon for serving

Directions:

Heat up a pan with the butter over medium heat, add applesauce, vanilla, eggs and maple syrup, stir well, take off heat and cool down. Add almond flour, cinnamon and baking powder, stir, pour in a cupcake pan, introduce in the oven at 350 degrees F and bake for 20 minutes. Take out of the oven, leave them to cool transfer to a platter, top with apple slices and sprinkle cinnamon before serving! Enjoy!

Nutrition: calories 110, fat 2, fiber 0, carbs 2, protein 4

Fruits and Orange Vinaigrette

It's such a pleasure to enjoy a delicious dessert!

Preparation time: 10 minutes
Cooking time: 15 minutes
Servings: 4

Ingredients:

- 1 cup orange juice
- 1 and ½ tablespoons sugar
- 1 and ½ tablespoons champagne vinegar
- 1 tablespoon olive oil
- 1 pound strawberries, halved
- 1 and ½ cups blueberries
- 1 peach, roughly chopped
- ¼ cup basil leaves, torn

Directions:

In a pot, mix orange juice with sugar and vinegar, stir, bring to a boil over medium high heat, simmer for 15 minutes, add oil, stir, take off heat and leave aside for a couple of minutes. In a bowl, mix blueberries with strawberries and peach wedges, add orange vinaigrettes, toss to coat, sprinkle basil on top and serve! Enjoy!

Nutrition: calories 10, fat 2, fiber 3, carbs 10, protein 2

Fruity Granita

It's a special and super easy to make dessert idea!

Preparation time: 6 hours and 10 minutes
Cooking time: 10 minutes
Servings: 3

Ingredients:

- 4 cups mango, peeled and cubed
- ¼ cup orange juice
- 6 tablespoons palm sugar
- 3 tablespoons lime juice
- A pinch of ground red pepper

Directions:

Put mango, orange juice, lime juice, sugar and red pepper in a small pot, stir, bring to a boil, reduce heat to low and simmer for 10 minutes. Leave this mixture aside to cool down a bit, transfer to a food processor, pulse a few times, strain into a container, introduce in the freezer and keep there for 6 hours scraping every hour. Enjoy!

Nutritional value: calories 80, fat 0, fiber 2, carbs 3, protein 2

Simple Grapefruit Granita

It's a wonderful dessert idea!

Preparation time: 4 hours and 20 minutes
Cooking time: 3 minutes
Servings: 3

Ingredients:

- 1 cup water
- 1 cup palm sugar
- ½ cup mint, chopped
- 64 ounces red grapefruit juice

Directions:

Put the water in a pan, bring to a boil over medium heat, add sugar, stir until it dissolves, take off heat, add mint, stir, cover and leave aside for 5 minutes Strain into a container, add grapefruit juice, stir, cover and freeze for 4 hours. Take out of the freezer 15 minutes before you serve it. Enjoy!

Nutrition: calories 80, fat 0, fiber 0, carbs 2, protein 1

Summer Berry Dessert

It's a good choice for a hot summer day!

Preparation time: 10 minutes
Cooking time: 5 minutes
Servings: 8

Ingredients:

- 1 and ½ cups blueberries
- 1 and ½ cups strawberries, cut in quarters
- 2 tablespoons cornstarch
- 3 tablespoons brown sugar
- 1 and ½ cups apple juice unsweetened
- Fat free vanilla yogurt for serving

Directions:

In a dish, mix blueberries with strawberries and 2 tablespoons sugar. Heat up a pot with the apple juice over medium high heat, add cornstarch, stir and boil for 2 minutes. Take sauce off heat, leave aside to cool down for 10 minutes, pour over fruit mix, add the rest of the sugar, stir gently, cover and keep in the fridge until your serve it. Spoon into dessert bowls and serve with fat free vanilla yogurt on top. Enjoy!

Nutrition: calories 100, fat 1, fiber 2, carbs 5, protein 2

Poached Plums

You don't need too many ingredients to make this dash diet dessert!

Preparation time: 10 minutes
Cooking time: 15 minutes
Servings: 4

Ingredients:

- 16 ripe plums, stoned and cut in halves
- 1 cup water
- ½ cup coconut sugar
- 5 cardamom pods, crushed

Directions:

Put water in a pot, add sugar and heat up over medium low heat. Add cardamom, bring to a boil and simmer for 10 minutes until sugar is dissolved. Add plums, stir gently, cover pot and cook for 5 minutes more. Leave plums aside to cool down before serving. Enjoy!

Nutrition: calories 90, fat 1, fiber 2, carbs 2, protein 3

Simple Baked Apples

This is a perfect dessert for you!

Preparation time: 10 minutes
Cooking time: 20 minutes
Servings: 4

Ingredients:

- 4 big apples, cored and tops cut off
- A handful raisins
- 1 tablespoon cinnamon
- 2 tablespoons honey to the taste

Directions:

Fill each apple with raisins, sprinkle cinnamon on them and drizzle honey at the end. Arrange all apples in a baking dish, introduce in the oven at 375 degrees F and bake for 20 minutes. Leave apples to cool down a bit before serving. Enjoy!

Nutrition: calories 100, fat 1, fiber 2, carbs 3, protein 3

Chestnut Jelly Cake

This dessert is one of our favorite ones!

Preparation time: 2 hours
Cooking time: 5 minutes
Servings: 3

Ingredients:
- 10 ounces chestnuts in syrup, chopped
- 1 teaspoon powdered agar agar
- 2 tablespoons azuki paste
- 7 ounces palm sugar
- 15 ounces water

Directions:

Put the water in a pot, bring to a boil over medium heat, add powdered agar and sugar, stir and cook for 5 minutes. Add chestnuts and azuki paste, stir until sugar dissolves, take off heat, pour into a container and keep in the freezer for 2 hours. Cut jelly into bars and serve as a tasty snack. Enjoy!

Nutrition: calories 140, fat 1, fiber 2, carbs 4, protein 5

Magical Lemon Cookies

Sit back and enjoy!

Preparation time: 2 hours and 10 minutes
Cooking time: 0 minutes
Servings: 10

Ingredients:
- 1/3 cup cashew butter
- 1 and ½ tablespoons coconut oil
- 2 tablespoons coconut butter
- 5 tablespoons lemon juice
- ½ teaspoon lemon zest, grated
- 1 tablespoons maple syrup

Directions:

In a bowl, mix cashew butter with coconut one, coconut oil, lemon juice, lemon zest and maple syrup and stir until you obtain a creamy mix. Line a cookie tray with some parchment paper, scoop 1 tablespoon of lemon cookie mix in each of the 10 pieces and freeze for 2 hours before serving. Enjoy!

Nutrition: calories 72, fat 1, fiber 0, carbs 2, protein 1

Conclusion

As you've recently discovered, a dash diet is not a restrictive one! You can enjoy various foods as long as you reduce your daily salt and bad fats intake.
This doesn't sound too hard to achieve, does it?

If you've decided that a dash diet is what you need today, then you must get your hands on a copy of this incredible cookbook!
It will help you get started with your new diet and it's going to become the most useful tool in the kitchen!

You will soon know how to make 150 of the most amazing and delicious dash diet recipes ever!
How can you still be hesitating? It's time to change your life forever and to start a dash diet!
Get this special cooking journal and start your new lifestyle as soon as possible!

Recipe Index

Made in the USA
Lexington, KY
02 March 2018